The
Little Book
of

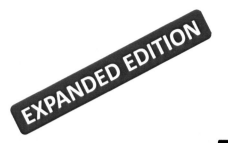

MENOPA**II**SE

Understanding the Biology and Management of Menopause

James R. Woods, Jr., M.D.

Elizabeth D. Warner, M.D.

Book Composition Coordinator: Jenna Brooks

Thank you to the following periFACTS® staff for their assistance with this book:
Yvonne Dougherty
Tamara Eis, MS, RN-BC
Kathryn Flynn, RNC, MSNP
Candace Galle, RN, BS, C-EFM
Ian Lawrence
Cynthia Slater
Patricia Therrien
Kalin Warshof, MS, RN, FNP-BC

CONTENTS

MENOPAUSE TRANSITION

HOT FLASHES

OBESITY AND CARDIOVASCULAR RISK

BONE HEALTH

ABOUT THE AUTHORS

James R. Woods, Jr., M.D. is Professor and past Chairman of the Department of Obstetrics and Gynecology at the University of Rochester School of Medicine and Dentistry in Rochester, New York. Dr. Woods has authored or co-authored over one hundred and forty articles on communication in medicine, maternal drug addiction, complications of pregnancy, and clinical research. Since 1991, he has been the editor-in-chief of the periFACTS® OB/GYN Academy, an international online educational program for obstetric and gynecologic care providers combining articles, clinical cases, grand rounds lectures, and teaching videos. In 1996, an endowed chair honoring Dr. Woods was established at the University of Rochester. He has been named in Best Doctors in America for many years. In 2010, Dr. Woods was honored by the American College of Obstetricians and Gynecologists with the Outstanding Service Award for District II for his "tireless efforts in the area of obstetric patient safety." In 2012, he received the lifetime achievement award from the District II American College of Obstetricians and Gynecologists. Dr. Woods has lectured extensively on communication in obstetrics and gynecology. He has pioneered strategies for transforming some of the most challenging clinical interactions with patients into extraordinary opportunities for compassionate communication between clinicians and their patients and family members.

Elizabeth D. Warner, M.D. received her undergraduate degree with honors from Cornell University (CALS) in 1975 and her medical degree from the University of Rochester School of Medicine and Dentistry (URMC), M.D. in 1979, member of Alpha Omega Alpha. She was a resident in the University of Rochester Strong Memorial Hospital Obstetrics and Gynecology program from 1979 to 1983. In August of 1983, she joined a private practice in Rochester, New York from which she retired in June of 2013. For approximately 20 years, she was the managing physician of this practice, and for the last ten years of her practice she had a particular interest in menopausal medicine. While in private practice, she held a teaching appointment at the University of Rochester Medical Center. She is currently Clinical Emeritus Professor of Obstetrics and Gynecology and she continues to teach medical students. She also has an interest in editing, and she is an active medical editor of periFACTS®, an online continuing education program for OB/GYN care providers. She is a Fellow of the American College of Obstetricians and Gynecologists (ACOG) and a member of the North American Menopause Society (NAMS), the American Society of Colposcopy and Cervical Pathology (ASCCP), and the American Urogynecologic Society (AUGS). She is married to a corporate health care attorney, now retired, and has adult identical twin sons.

PREFACE

Considerable confusion exists among women and their care providers regarding the biology of the menopause. Once considered a one year problem for some women, (at a time when premenstrual syndrome was considered just a mood disorder) menopause is now recognized as starting in the 40s, and for some, extending into the 70s. As such, in the past decade, this important field of women's health has emerged as factual, structured, and formal. Why do these menopausal symptoms appear? How long do they last? What is their impact on personal lifestyle and business economics? And what safe measures can be employed to modify them? In recent years scientists have contributed significant information as to the etiologies of hot flashes, mood swings, memory loss, vaginal dryness, loss of libido, bone and heart health. Yet so little of this information is known to care providers who daily must care for these challenged women as the U.S. population ages.

These essays address the role of inflammation as the underlying cause of most of the menopause symptoms, the biologic impact that loss of estrogen plays in this process, and the role that hormone replacement serves to reduce these symptoms. Care providers in women's health now have a responsibility to embrace care of menopausal women with the same level of professionalism as they apply to obstetrics and gynecology of younger women. Our understanding of the biology of menopause now make both possible. Moreover, women receiving gynecologic care, by becoming more educated about menopause, can engage with their care providers in a meaningful conversation.

GENERAL DISCUSSION

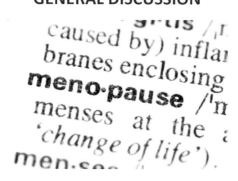

INTRODUCTION

The term "menopause" often generates a great deal of misunder-standing and frustration among those women who enter that chapter of their lives.

Why me? Why have the years when I was having children been so well orchestrated for the preservation of the species, only to leave me feeling like this? When I see my doctor, my first thoughts are "What has happened to my memory, why am I gaining weight, why is my skin drying up, what is bone loss, why is intercourse painful, in fact why do I not care for sex at all and why do I go from urinary tract infection, to vaginal yeast infection, to other infections around my vagina, and then back to urinary tract infection? What are these bursting moments of hot flashes, why do my moods swing so widely, and what are these new awkward aches? Why does my doctor talk to me about my cardiac risks when fear of breast cancer is my mountain to climb, and what are my options for management of these problems? If my doctor talks about hormonal management, I am really confused regarding what are bioidentical hormones, should I go on hormones and for how long, and what are the differences between the estrogen patch and the pill?"

These are some of the questions that women from the ages of 40 years to 70 years bring to the primary care physician's and gynecologist's office each day. Are these women looking for a cure? Are they looking to understand what is happening to their bodies? In general, yes. For most of them, when presented with current information regarding the biology of menopause, they are willing to accept the fact that this is just another phase of a normal life. Yet it is the obligation of the primary care physician and gynecologist to help women find solutions for these issues.

What is clear is that the term, menopause, once considered that one year in which a woman no longer has a menstrual period, today is thought of as a more comprehensive and lengthy part of life. We now understand that changes in hormonal production from the ovaries usually begins between years 40 and 45 leading to the mean age of 51 years for that final menstrual period. More importantly, that one year without menstruation is only part of a process extending from around 40 years to 70 years. In that period of nearly 30 years, scientists have helped us to understand that there are specific biological events that explain most of the symptoms that women describe, including mood swings, hot flashes, pain of intercourse, loss of libido, skin dryness, changes in bone structure, breast cancer risk, cardiovascular health, and aging. Yet every woman goes through this process in a manner unique only to herself.

In the following essays, we will provide short discussions regarding specific aspects of menopause. To accomplish this task, we are drawing from information generated by scientists in this field, since it is now clear that our current and future knowledge of the symptoms women encounter in this phase of their lives can be explained by specific biological events. And it is alterations in these same biological events that encourage us to return to the basic roles of hormones in the body, how these hormones change as menopause is approached, and how the benefits and risks of the many options for hormonal management participate in the care of women's health.

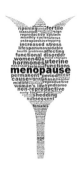

THE PUBLIC FACE OF MENOPAUSE

Recently, *Menopause the Musical* played to a full house in Rochester, New York. After opening in 2001 in a 76-seat theater in Orlando, Florida, it now shows worldwide and incorporates 25 popular songs from the 1960s to the 1980s. With clever word arrangements provided by four outstanding vocalists, it addresses most of the common personal menopausal issues women struggle to understand. Everyone who has had the opportunity to see this musical knows how brilliant it is. Yet, as I looked around the room, I was impressed by the large number of men in the audience. And with musical humor, this singular entertainment event has become the poster child of a major change that is occurring in our society; the public conversation of a once forbidden topic.

Have we elevated the biology of menopause to parallel public efforts in diabetes, heart disease, and cancer? Not yet. We are more comfortable with the topic of women's health than in the days of the twin beds of *I Love Lucy*. But have we made meaningful progress? The media certainly have desensitized us with nonstop sex and violence. How many magazines displayed in grocery stores offer lead articles suggesting "100 Ways That Your Man Can Make Your Sex Better." Or, "What Women Want From Their Toy Boy." Yet, the personal and intimate discussions that women should have with their partners and their care providers about their own bodies have been off limits until recently.

As with any topic involving the female body, there are issues that are personal to the woman and those that impact directly on the partnership. Menopause medicine today is elevating women's medicine to a new level. Today's caregiver must be educated in the management of mood swings, memory loss, hot flashes, skin changes, pain during intercourse, incontinence, and breast, bone, and cardiac health.

Pain during intercourse (dyspareunia), however, is possibly the most private of menopausal issues a couple must deal with. Lower levels of estrogen lead to vaginal dryness and tissue changes, which can cause painful intercourse. Why do I say "couple?" Why were there so many men at *Menopause the Musical*? Menopause is not just a woman's problem; it embraces the entire relationship, and men realize that. Loss of intimacy leads to struggles with depression. Mood swings accelerate her depression. And with those changes comes a further deterioration of the relationship. Witness the husband and wife who present for an initial consult. He says, "Please, can you help us? She has no energy, she never laughs anymore, and we no longer have sex." In that same safe environment, she says, "What has happened to me? In my forties I had lots of energy, pep, was full of fun, and loved sex. Now I don't even know who I am. Please help me."

Today, we as care providers benefit from the knowledge that scientists have provided to help us to become better educators in the field of menopause. And from our heightened awareness of the couple's needs, we can advance the importance of diet and exercise, weight loss, the role of alternative medicines, and finally, hormonal management. The menopause pendulum is swinging in a positive direction, and women and their families will benefit. Knowledge is power.

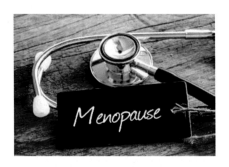

UNDERSTANDING MENOPAUSE (AT THE MOST BASIC LEVEL)

Recent advances in the biology of menopause have helped clarify the importance of female hormones in women's overall health. Improved patient education that allows women to engage in formal conversations with their care providers helps clinicians to individualize menopause management for their patients. In essence, while menopause is a complex process, it can be understood at a basic level by viewing it simply as a process of hormone withdrawal. And the hormone of most importance is estradiol, cyclically produced in large amounts by the ovaries during the reproductive years, reflecting the high numbers of eggs that rapidly decrease in number as one approaches menopause.

During reproductive years, estradiol is critical for menstrual cycles and pregnancy. More recently, scientists have found that during these years, estradiol also has an anti-inflammatory action, preventing immune cells and visceral fat cells from activating certain inflammatory cytokines, including interleukin 1, interleukin 6 and tumor necrosis factor alpha. Yet, it is these same inflammatory proteins that our scientists have linked to essentially all of the more common menopausal symptoms, such as hot flashes, mood swings, memory loss, dry skin, vaginal dryness, low libido, bone breakdown, and cardiovascular risk.

In the past, menopause was considered one full year without any menstruation. We now know that in the several months-to-years leading up to that one year without menstruation, the ovaries gradually become more resistant to hormone control from the brain. This window in time, previously known as perimenopause, now is formally termed the Menopause Transition. Women may only recognize this by encountering irregular menstrual periods. During this interval, however, fluctuations of estradiol from the ovaries begin to allow immune cells and visceral fat cells to release low levels of these inflammatory cytokines into the bloodstream. The result is that these women may begin to experience early menopause symptoms, even though they still are having irregular periods.

The menopause transition represents more than simply the emergence of early menopausal symptoms. This period is associated with significant increases in visceral fat, cholesterol and triglycerides; thickening of the walls of carotid arteries; weight gain; and reduced physical activity.

During menopause, estradiol essentially becomes undetectable in the blood. One would expect that all women, therefore, would experience the classic symptoms of menopause, but that is not so. Despite low levels of estradiol, women entering menopause will differ in how they perceive absence of estradiol. Some will experience only minimal or mild symptoms, while others will feel that they are overwhelmed by new, distressing symptoms. The duration of these symptoms also differs among women. For some women, symptoms will pass within a few years. Recent longitudinal studies now indicate that for other women, symptoms of menopause may last well into their 60s or even 70s.

Scientists have helped clarify the biology of menopause. Clinicians now better understand the range of responses women experience during menopause. These two revelations have matured the field of menopause medicine. Some women will find that education alone is sufficient. Others will need the education to enter into a conversation regarding management. Whether it is through therapeutic listening, complementary and alternative medicines, or hormone replacement, menopause medicine now is a rich, mature, and established field of medicine. Women have always known that menopause is real. The medical community still is working to improve each woman's menopausal life.

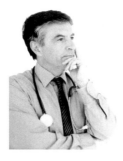
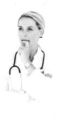

WHY IS MENOPAUSE MANAGEMENT NOT BETTER UNDERSTOOD BY OB/GYN CARE PROVIDERS?

Today, menopause management as a finite field of medicine is a product of many laboratory and clinical studies targeted at understanding the biology of menopause and the impact of hormonal and non-hormonal treatments. Why, then, do women in the menopausal transition or in menopause itself often confront a medical community that is either not aware of or is even indifferent to the challenges they face?

The concept of menopause is not new. Symptoms of menopause in midlife were observed in women as far back as the time of Aristotle. By 1921, the term "menopause" gave this time of life a name. However, women's psychosocial issues were slow to gain recognition, perhaps because gynecologic care was provided by mostly male physicians in an era of paternalistic medicine. Evidence the debate in the 1970s as to whether premenstrual dysphoria actually existed. The concept that symptoms of menopause might begin months or years before that one year without a menstrual period (officially called menopause) or that the symptoms for some women might last well into their 70s was not discussed.

In 1968, Robert Wilson, a gynecologist in New York City, published *Feminine Forever* advocating that menopause was a discrete time of life and was treatable. In his own words, "The often-severe suffering of my menopausal patients made me regard menopause as a serious medical condition endangering the health and happiness of any woman...In the vast majority of cases the distressing bodily changes following menopause are reversible through estrogen treatment." Unfortunately, by portraying menopause as a "disease to be treated," he inflamed the feminist movement, which at that time was advocating menopause as a natural transition in life to be tolerated and even embraced.

It was out of that debate that in 1992 the Women's Health Initiative was funded by the National Institutes of Health (NIH) to study hormone replacement and its potential preventive actions. Those results and subsequent study-analyses, fueled by the pharmaceutical industry, spawned a wide range of treatments for menopause. Around that same time, in 1989, the North American Menopause Society was formed, bringing together scientists and physicians in OB/GYN and general medicine with a goal to "promote the health and quality of life of all women during midlife and beyond through an understanding of menopause and healthy aging."

Even with these efforts, why do women patients still ask, "Why is menopause not better understood by care providers?" Here are four possible answers. 1. Formal training in OB/GYN is usually clinic based, involving younger patients with a focus on obstetrics, contraception, and sexually transmitted infections. 2. The practice of OB/GYN demands that the practitioner acquires a wide range of surgical skills for managing obstetric care and gynecologic surgery. Menopause management is not dominated by the requirement of manual surgical skills. 3. Menopause management in the office is time-intensive in an era when insurance reimbursement rewards procedures and shorter visits with higher numbers of patients seen. 4. Menopause management requires more individualization of education and treatment, which is, by itself, a higher level skill in medicine. This form of practice is more trial and error than much of medicine and requires patience by clinician and patient, an emotion which is often in short supply in our world of short attention spans.

Is there a brighter future for menopause care? Efforts are underway to improve research, therapeutics, and gynecologic care to address the needs of educated menopausal women. As more women care providers age and become more interested in menopause medicine, patients will benefit. In addition, women themselves will bring about change as they become better educated about menopause management. Menopause is a time of life, NOT a disease.

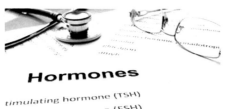

Hormones

CLARIFYING THE TERMS "BIOIDENTICAL HORMONES" AND "COMPOUNDED HORMONES"

The terms "bioidentical hormones," "compounded hormones," and "compounded bioidentical hormones" often are used improperly in conversations between care providers and patients. But the fact that these medications even exist is a tribute to the evolving story of hormone development.

It was Claude Bernard, French physiologist, who first noted that glands in the body produced substances that could affect other organs. Then, in 1906, secretions from the ovaries were found to produce estrus, and the term "estrogen" was born. By 1930, various placental and ovarian hormones had been identified and, in 1938, researchers reported that a complex of estrogens could be isolated from pregnant mare urine which they called Premarin®. The Canadian-based pharmaceutical firm, Ayerst, McKenna, and Harrison (later to become Wyeth Pharmaceuticals) began producing Premarin®. Premarin®, however, was not a pure estrogen but instead contained a wide range of different estrogens including estrone sulfate (50% to 60%), equilin sulfate (22% to 32%), and less than 5% estradiol sulfate, the principle estrogen made by the ovary during reproductive life. Premarin® became available for clinical use in 1941 and received Federal Drug Administration (FDA) approval in 1942.

Premarin® contains a range of estrogens and other hormones. Following intestinal absorption of the hormone pill, there is a first pass through the liver with release of a wide range of other hormones and clotting factors, which led researchers to seek an alternative source for pure estrogens. The solution was the development of bioidentical hormones.

Bioidentical hormones are produced in the laboratory from plants (wild yams, cactus, or soy), but, when modified, the structures and functions of these hormones are identical to those of the hormones made by the body. While wild yams had been used since the 18th century to treat menstrual cramps, in the 1950s scientists identified diosgenin, the phytoestrogen in plant roots, which could be chemically converted to such hormones as progesterone, estrogen, testosterone, DHEA, and cortisol.

The bioidentical hormone story, therefore, starts in the laboratory where the phytoestrogens are extracted from plants. Compounding pharmacies and pharmaceutical companies obtain those same bioidentical hormone products from the same chemical laboratory companies, but their paths then diverge. The pharmaceutical companies prepare their products (pills, gels, creams, or patches) under strict FDA regulations. The compounding pharmacies take the same bioidentical hormone preparations and develop them into their own preparations. The advantage of the compounding pharmacies is that they can tailor the dosages delivered to the patient, while the pharmaceutical companies have a more restricted dose range of hormones they can offer on the market. However, while the pharmaceutical companies are under strict safety rules, vis-á-vis the FDA, compounding pharmacies must report to their state pharmacy boards only. There are many reputable compounding pharmacies. However, the most recent cases of meningitis following injection of tainted steroids from a compounding pharmacy have resulted in a proposed bill in Congress to provide the FDA with more oversight over compounding pharmacies.

Proper menopause management requires that the care provider be aware of the various indications, preparations, benefits, and risks of hormone therapy. Armed with that knowledge, he or she becomes an effective educator and advisor of women going through menopause.

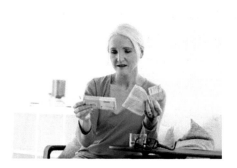

WAS THE WOMEN'S HEALTH INITITIATIVE GOOD OR BAD FOR WOMEN'S HEALTH?

Most women are familiar with the Women's Health Initiative (WHI), the largest randomized controlled trial to date, which was sponsored by the National Institute of Health (NIH) to evaluate the role of hormone therapy in menopause to protect cardiovascular and bone health. Begun in 1991 as a proposed 15-year study, women in menopause with a uterus were randomized to take orally either a placebo or PremPro®, a combination of Premarin®, a conjugated equine estrogen (CEE) and medroxyprogesterone, a synthetic version of progesterone. Women with a hysterectomy were given either CEE alone or placebo. In part, this $725 million study was intended to resolve the controversy over whether menopause should be embraced as a natural transition in life, a position taken by the feminist movement at the time, or, as proposed by such books as *Feminine Forever* (Pocket Books, NY, 1968), that menopause was a hormone deficiency totally preventable with hormone therapy.

In 2002, the entire study was abruptly stopped due to a statistical increase in breast cancer and stroke and no apparent benefit for reducing cardiovascular risk. This bold action by the NIH prompted the New York Times article entitled, "Hormone Replacement Study: A Shock to the Medical System." As one physician later wrote, "I may have taken my last pill this morning." By 2003, there was a precipitous reduction in hormone prescriptions, ushering in a decade of menopausal women without hormone support. But was the WHI study done correctly?

The purpose of hormone replacement in menopause is to compensate for the lack of estrogen, primarily estradiol, of which 95% is produced by the ovaries during the reproductive years. The role of a progestin is to duplicate progesterone, produced cyclically by the premenopausal ovaries, whose sole purpose is to prevent overstimulation of the uterine lining by estradiol.

Three aspects of the WHI deserve closer scrutiny: the age of the women in the study, the choice of the hormones used, and the significance of the statistical risk.

With an average age of 63 years, many of these women participating in the study may already have had vascular damage from age-related changes, thus increasing their risks for cardiovascular events. The average age of menopause in the United States is 51 years.

In the WHI, Premarin®, derived from the urine of pregnant mares (Pre-mar-in) contains ten different estrogens but almost no estradiol, the most powerful of the body's estrogens. Taken as an estrogen pill, it is absorbed in the intestine, with a "first pass" through the liver, increasing production of many clotting factors. This explains the increased incidence of stroke in both arms of the study. Conversely, transdermal estrogen does not stimulate these clotting factors. Medroxyprogesterone was used as the progestin. This is a synthetic chemical version of progesterone. Women on PremPro® did show a statistical increase in breast cancer. Yet, those women with a hysterectomy, and therefore taking Premarin® only, showed a reduction in breast cancer mortality. Was it the progestin? Recent data suggests that medroxyprogesterone in breast tissue may alter hormone receptors adjacent to the estrogen receptors, thus increasing the risks of estrogen-stimulated cancers.

Applying statistical risk to clinical risk also is a challenge. In the WHI, out of 10,000 person-years, there were seven more cardiac events, eight more strokes, eight more pulmonary emboli, and eight more breast cancers. The WHI frightened women (a negative), but it laid the groundwork for improved menopausal care (a positive). Today, there is a growing sense that if women are started on hormone replacement in their late 40s or early 50s and are administered pure estradiol by a patch or cream and pure progesterone, that the original hypotheses of the WHI might have been better served.

◫◫

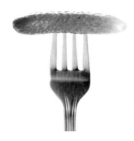

SPICE, PICKLES FOR LEG CRAMPS. CAN IT BE THAT SIMPLE?

Most people have experienced muscle cramps, usually in the form of leg cramps. Surveys suggest that one-third of adults over 60 years old and half of those over 80 experience muscle cramps, some reporting symptoms for ten years or longer. They strike without warning, often in the night, and usually, slowly respond as one keeps the extremity involved on stretch until the cramps subside. Extrapolating from the experiences of athletes who get exercise-induced cramps and people with peripheral vascular disease who get activity-related cramps, one would assume that muscle cramps must represent muscle fatigue, electrolyte imbalance, or tissue ischemia. Yet, many muscle cramps occur temporally distant from any physical exertion and often when hydration is not an issue. And for many athletes, hydration or electrolyte solutions have failed to prevent or adequately treat their occurrence.

Can your palate fix your leg cramps? The Wall Street Journal (WSJ) usually is not one's initial go-to medical source for explaining complex health issues. Yet, on July 11, 2016, Matthew Futterman reported on the unique pursuit by neurobiologist, biophysicist, and Noble prizewinner, Rod MacKinnon, and his colleague, neurobiologist, Bruce Bean, to rethink this common yet poorly understood phenomenon. If dehydration and electrolyte abnormalities were not the cause, could it be that overstimulation of motor neurons serving the muscles could explain a muscle cramp? Further, they hypothesized that introducing a strong sensory input might inhibit or even block the motor output affecting the muscle. After a series of studies and with input from athletes, the researchers concluded that a spicy drink might provide the strong sensory input they were seeking. Since the ameliorating effect of this strong sensory input occurs within seconds to minutes after the spicy drink is ingested, the sensory trigger must originate in the palate or posterior esophagus.

MacKinnon and Bean found that stimulation of the transient receptor potential ion channels (TRP) and acid-sensing ion channels (ASIC) with strong spices or acids (acetic acid in vinegar in pickle juice) in the palate and esophagus cause a sensory overload that can then block the motor neuron overstimulation which causes the muscle to cramp. It turns out that there are several kinds of TRP channels that respond to different molecular stimuli including acid, pungent spices (ginger, allicin in garlic, and cinnamon), and hot spices (capsaicin in chili peppers and allyl isothiocyanate in wasabi). Drs. MacKinnon and Bean subsequently helped start a new company producing a liquid drink containing ginger, cinnamon, and capsicum to prevent and treat muscle cramps.

Further validation of this phenomenon resulted from other studies of athletes. In one study, on two separate days one week apart, mildly dehydrated male athletes were subjected each day to two episodes of muscle cramps induced by tibial nerve stimulation with each episode separated by 30 minutes. On the second study day, the athletes were given either deionized water or dill pickle juice immediately after the second cramp. While on the first study day, the duration of the two cramp episodes was similar, on the second study day, the muscle cramp duration for those athletes given pickle juice was shorter (49 seconds) than for those given water (85 seconds), yet no changes in blood chemistries were seen in either group. In a follow-up study of mildly dehydrated athletes who were administered pickle juice or mustard (a second spicy ingredient that some have found effective against muscle cramps), none of the study participants demonstrated any changes in blood chemistries. This provided further evidence that any muscle cramp-blocking effect of these spices is localized.

Anecdotes on cures and prevention of muscle cramps abound. Midwifery literature is replete with advice that pregnant women should ingest pickle juice to prevent muscle cramps. I add my own personal experience. In the midst of a 3 a.m. muscle cramp, after having read this article, I stumbled to the refrigerator where I found a large jar of dill pickles. Quickly pouring pickle juice into a small glass, I reluctantly, but quickly, drank it. Within 30 seconds, the cramp was completely gone. Later that day, I recounted this episode to one of my patients, a 77-year-old woman whose husband is undergoing dialysis. She smiled at my story only to relate that during dialysis treatment her husband suffered severe muscle cramps until a patient in the next cubical told him to "eat a pickle." He has religiously employed this advice and has not had a single dialysis-induced muscle cramp since.

The health field is portrayed as an impenetrable forest of facts too complicated for the average person to understand. In this case, the keen eye and inquisitive approach by two esteemed scientists may have explained and confirmed the folklore cure for one of the most common yet irritating events in life.

⬚⬚

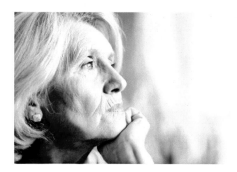

I'M GETTING OLDER...AM I STILL RELEVANT?

Only you can make yourself unhappy. That is, perhaps, a non-psychological layman's interpretation of cognitive behavioral therapy, the concept that while you cannot control all of the slings and arrows the outside world throws at you that may make you question your worth, only you can control how you react to them.

Most of us at one time or another question if we have value. Am I important to others? Does anyone really need me? These moments more likely descend upon us at times of personal crisis. Perhaps because of the death of my loved one, I am left alone. My partner has had an affair. My child with bipolar disorder is failing in school. I am likely to lose my job. Or my cancer is returning. During those moments, the feelings of helplessness and even worthlessness can be all-consuming. "Why should I get out of bed this morning?" Or worse, "Will anyone care if I get out of bed this morning?"

In a gynecology practice focused on menopause, a transition-filled, existential time of questioning for many women, these questions often are the real substance of the visit. The reason for the visit may be documented as "a urinary tract infection" or "a vaginal bump." Yet, these may not be the real issues challenging a woman's life. When asked how life is in general, the truth may be revealed reluctantly at first. But, with encouragement, a full conversation may follow with the real struggles that the woman is encountering. She is seeking help from her gynecologist for emotional suffering or a quest for meaning: "Am I valued?" Said differently, "Am I relevant?"

But being relevant means many things. It might be that you work to generate a salary to pay the bills. But, it also may be volunteer work that helps others. Or, the weekly phone call to connect with your granddaughter who lives in another state. Or, even mowing the lawn for your elderly neighbor.

In our role as gynecologists, we are uniquely positioned to really listen to what a woman is trying to communicate and to provide a human response. One simple step is to ask her to make a list of events of which she is proud or people for whom she is grateful. Her first response may be, "I probably will not have anything to say." Of course, the natural counter would be, "If you really feel that you are unworthy or have little to be grateful for, then your page will be blank." But, every woman has something or someone in her life that engenders pride or gratitude. This exercise may seem too basic for such a serious condition as depression. Yet, as a first step, it often generates pages of positive information that can facilitate a path to healing, not a blank sheet.

Life is brief, and the time we have has meaning, but only if we, within ourselves, recognize those contributions we have made toward it that make us who we are. We, as gynecologists, have the privilege of sharing in this search for meaning.

HORMONE BIOLOGY

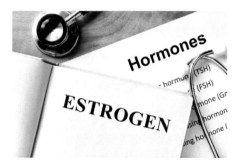

THE STORY OF ESTROGEN: NOT JUST YOUR MOTHER'S HORMONE

The story of the history of estrogen illustrates the historical progression of medical knowledge, from laboratory and clinical observation, through basic and clinical experimentation, to current successful medical management, an interesting marriage of empiricism and technology.

Our bodies efficiently make our natural hormones. Cholesterol from our diet is converted into a family of progesterones, which then become our androgens, such as testosterone, androstenedione, and dehydroepiandrosterone (DHEA). Androgens are important since they are the substrate for all of the estrogens in our body. The ovaries alone convert testosterone to estradiol (E2), the most powerful of the estrogens. Fat cells can convert androstenedione to other weaker estrogens, including estrone (E1), only 40% as active as estradiol, and estriol (E3), only 10% as active as estradiol. Since menopausal symptoms seem to arise with falling estrogen levels, estrogen has been sought as treatment of these symptoms.

How did estrogen come to dominate the discussion of menopause? In the late 1800s, knowledge of hormones was nonexistent, and medical decision-making was based solely on empirical observation. As a prelude to the discovery of other hormones, in the mid-1850s,

Claude Bernard demonstrated that glands had internal secretions that could influence other organs. In 1897, ovarian extract was found to be effective for the treatment of menopausal hot flushing. Then, in 1906, secretions from the ovaries were shown to produce estrus (cyclic sexual activity in non-human females) and the term "estrogen" was born, derived from the Greek oistros (mad desire) and gennan (to produce). Yet, it was not until 1929 that estrogen as a hormone was isolated.

The first commercial preparation of estrogen began as an estrogen complex extracted from placentas called Emmenin, which was used to treat dysmenorrhea. The pharmaceutical company Ayerst, McKennen, and Harrison, Ltd. then developed Emmenin as the first oral female sex hormone. In 1938, an article appeared describing a similar collection of substances from pregnant mare urine (PMU). That publication led to the commercial production of PMU in 1939, at which point it was renamed Premarin® (pregnant-mare-urine). Premarin® contained at least ten estrogens, the dominant ones being estrone (50% to 60%) and equilin (22.5% to 32.5%) with less than 5% estradiol. Premarin® became commercially available in the United States (U.S.) in 1942. By 1992, Premarin® was the number one prescribed drug in the U.S., with sales exceeding $1 billion in 1997.

This changed drastically in July of 2002, when the release of results from the Women's Health Initiative (WHI) abruptly altered women's attitudes toward hormone replacement therapy (HRT). A documented statistical increase in breast cancer and stroke by menopausal women taking PremPro® (Premarin® and Provera®) led to many women abruptly stopping HRT with a resulting significant drop in prescriptions. This also fueled the search for a safer delivery system for estrogen.

Today, all of the major estrogens except Premarin® are derived from plants or synthesized denovo and are bioidentical hormones, i.e., identical in structure and function to the body's own estrogens. Most of these can be delivered transdermally or intravaginally. Why is this an advantage? All oral estrogens undergo a first pass through the liver via the portal system before entering the general circulation. This leads to a rise in inflammatory and procoagulant markers with a resultant increased risk of venous thrombosis. Transdermal estrogen significantly reduces these risks by entering the bloodstream directly, bypassing the liver. Progesterone, which is part of HRT given to decrease uterine cancer risk with estrogen alone, can be given intravaginally, transdermally, or perhaps via intrauterine device. It turns out that women without a uterus in the WHI, who therefore did not need the progesterone component of HRT, did not have a greater risk of cardiovascular accident (CVA) or myocardial infarction (MI). However, this was greatly downplayed at the time of the released data in 2002.

Improvements in the delivery and understanding of estrogen's role in perimenopausal and postmenopausal women, including risks and benefits, have led to a better quality of life for women as their lifespan continues to increase. With further research and clinical study, this should only continue to improve.

〇〇

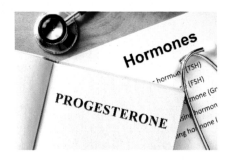

FROM MENARCHE TO MENOPAUSE: THE STORY OF PROGESTERONE

The hormone progesterone frequently is discussed with regard to menstruation, fertility, pregnancy, and contraception during reproductive years or in the context of hormone replacement therapy (HRT) with estrogen in menopause. Women, however, often have questions as to the nature of "natural" progesterone as compared with a progestin, which is a synthetic version, or why the route of administration may at times create different reactions, risks, and benefits.

Progesterone's role in the menstrual cycle is well understood. The reproductive cycle is controlled by a small group of neurons in the hypothalamus called the KNDy neurons (kisspepsin, neurokinin B, and dynorphin), which become active at puberty. Under their control, gonadotrophin-releasing hormone neurons in the hypothalamus activate the pituitary to release follicle-stimulating hormone (FSH) and luteinizing hormone (LH) to stimulate the ovaries to advance follicle development. During the follicular or growth phase of the menstrual cycle, estrogen secretion from the ovaries acts on the endometrium, the lining of the uterus, to thicken it by converting short, straight, narrow glands in the decidua to long, tortuous glands. A spike of LH leads to extrusion of the ovum (ovulation). The fimbria of the fallopian tubes captures the ovum and, if sperm are available, fertilization can follow. The ovarian site of ovulation, now called the corpus luteum, begins to produce progesterone to further develop the endometrium in order to maintain the anticipated early pregnancy. With failure of fertilization, estrogen and progesterone levels fall, decidual ischemia develops, and menses results.

Discerning the biologic effect of progesterone can first be traced to R. deGraaf (1672) and later to L.A. Prenent and G. Born (1898). Others, in the early 1900s, wrote of the effects of secretions from the corpus luteum upon the endometrium. Then, in 1929, G.W. Corner and W.A. Allen demonstrated the importance of the corpus luteum for maintaining the early pregnancy.

But understanding the structure of the hormone and not just its actions was achieved by R.E. Marker at The Pennsylvania State College (later University) who started with Sarsasapogenin, a plant steroid isolated from Sarsaparilla. He produced progesterone in a three-step chemical process that became known as the "Marker Degradation." Using Sarsasapogenin and its laboratory manipulation, however, was very expensive. The next historical step was to utilize the Beth root from the lily family to produce Diogenin, a compound which previously had been isolated by the Japanese from a yam of the Dioscorea family. Then, in 1941, Marker learned of a plant called Cabeza de Negro, also of the Dioscorea family, existing in Vercruz, Mexico. When no United States company was interested, Marker returned to Mexico and dried ten tons of it to make 3 kilograms of progesterone. Through the 1940s, Marker formed or joined several companies as other investigators began taking the lead to economically develop progesterone production from plants.

Synthetic progestins, in contrast, were birthed in a laboratory. Scientists, applying techniques used to convert testosterone to estrone and estradiol, coupled with additional known chemical steps, produced norethindrone. Norethindrone, a progestin, is one of the two active components (along with an estrogen) of the first oral contraceptive pills (OCP). Later generations of progestins in OCPs and HRT formulations differed from each other in their affinities for estrogen, androgen, and progesterone receptors with resulting differing side effects. With the ability to inhibit ovulation, alone or in combination with estrogens, progestins now are accepted as critical components of oral contraceptives, intrauterine devices, and progesterone contraceptive implants.

The role of progesterone and progestins in menopause medicine as part of HRT, however, has been more controversial. Progesterone was not always a part of HRT. The effectiveness of estrogen to reduce menopausal symptoms led the Food and Drug Administration (FDA) to approve diethylstilbestrol (DES) in 1941 and Premarin® in 1942. As a result, estrogen use soared in the 1960s and early 1970s until mid-1970 when reports of estrogen-related endometrial hyperplasia and cancer began to appear. The addition of a progestin to counter the stimulatory effect of estrogen on the endometrium resulted in PremPro®, a combination of Premarin®, a conjugated group of estrogens derived from the urine of pregnant mares and medroxyprogesterone acetate, a progestin. This product was employed in the Women's Health Initiative (WHI), a study with the intent to prove the efficacy of menopausal hormones for bone and heart health. Instead it demonstrated a small increased risk of breast cancer, a shocking result that was not found in the second arm of that study that only employed Premarin® for women who did not have a uterus. The use of all HRT plummeted after 2002 when the results were published and the study prematurely stopped. Today, current thinking is that the responsible agent was the progestin when combined with Premarin®.

Modern HRT requires that a menopausal woman with a uterus who is on estrogen must take some type of progesterone. While progestins are still used by some, oral micronized progesterone has become the standard. Some have used a daily dose of 100 mg. Others use 200 mg for 14 days at the end of every three months. But, premenstrual-like discomfort often is described as a side effect of this higher dose. Because oral progesterone must be absorbed by the intestine and has a "first pass" through the liver, this route often is bypassed by using progesterone as a vaginal suppository. Studies of infertility patients on progesterone indicate that the vaginal route is a more effective way to deliver progesterone to the uterus.

The science of hormones continues to have its champions and its critics. Still, progress is being made as scientists and clinicians combine laboratory and clinical studies to improve women's health.

〇〇

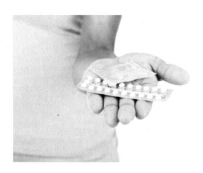

THE PILL OR THE PATCH: ARE ALL ESTROGENS THE SAME?

Picture this scenario. You are 55 years old, three years into menopause, with hot flashes, mood swings, and vaginal dryness and pain on intercourse. Your care provider suggests hormone replacement therapy (HRT). However, he recalls that in 2002, the Women's Health Initiative (WHI) reported that of 10,000 women-years, HRT produced 18 more women with blood clots, eight more with stroke, and seven more with heart attacks than those not on hormones. You have a family history of blood clots. You hesitate, "Is this for me?"

Advances in hormone therapy have helped explain many of the adverse vascular outcomes of the WHI. This study compared women on no hormones to those on PremPro®, made up of Premarin®, which is a mixture of estrogens from extracts of pregnant mare's urine, and Provera®, which is medroxyprogesterone acetate, a synthetic derivative of progesterone. For women with a prior hysterectomy, Premarin® alone was given. Both hormone-treated groups showed increases in blood clots and stroke. Why?

Our blood is designed to deliver oxygen and nutrition to our cells within a careful balance of biologic factors that normally keep our blood "fluid" under the influence of protein C, protein S, and thrombomodulin. When bleeding occurs, substances released at the site of bleeding activate events to form a clot which eventually must be broken down (lysed) to restore circulation.

How is this done? When hemorrhage occurs, platelets initially drawn there by release of von Willebrand factor and collagen from the injury site plug the defect. Then, at the site of injury, other tissue factors convert prothrombin to thrombin. In turn, thrombin converts fibrinogen, normally soluble in our blood, into a mesh to form a stable clot. Once hemorrhage is stopped, plasmin, produced by release of tissue plasminogen activator, begins to dissolve the clot and restore circulation.

So how does estrogen influence this process? It seems that when Premarin® is ingested as a pill, it is absorbed in the gut and then passes through the liver. This "first pass" in the liver produces a range of other steroids, but also may increase the risk of clotting. Some have proposed that this "first pass" through the liver alters the balance of prostacycline (a vasodilator) and thromboxane A2 (a vasoconstrictor) or reduces the effectiveness of protein C to keep blood fluid.

In contrast, transdermal estrogen patches, which were first studied in 1997, deliver pure estradiol slowly through the skin that is then absorbed directly into the bloodstream. Because of this slow, steady, delivery rate, which to some extent mimics how the ovaries functioned during reproductive years, a lower sustained estrogen dose achieves biologic effects equivalent to those of higher dose estrogen pills. While studies are not as numerous as with oral pills, a consistent conclusion is that transdermal estrogen does not involve a "first pass" and does not change the normal balance of coagulation and anticoagulation factors, thus decreasing blood clotting risk.

In a recent article in the national journal, *Menopause*, a thorough review concluded that transdermal estrogen does not increase blood clotting risk as does oral estrogen. Perhaps HRT is for you but in a more modern form.

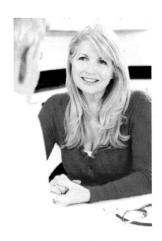

PROGRESS IN SAFETY OF HORMONE DELIVERY

Women depend on their reproductive hormones in many ways. During the reproductive years, estradiol, the most powerful of the estrogen family, is produced largely by the ovaries. While it is important for menstrual cycles and pregnancy, we now know that estradiol plays a key role in keeping your body in an uninflamed state. Estradiol accomplishes this by depressing the ability of your fat cells and immune cells to activate a number of inflammatory proteins that are linked to many of the menopausal symptoms women describe. Even in the several years leading up to that one year without a menstrual period (a window of time called the Menopause Transition), fluctuations in ovarian production of estradiol cause these inflammatory proteins to become functional. These fluctuations explain why mood swings, hot flashes, skin changes, and loss of libido may be encountered, even as the menstrual periods still are occurring.

If reductions in estradiol lead to many of these menopausal symptoms, should reintroducing estradiol into the body early in menopause combat these changes? Progress in safety of hormone delivery has helped here.

In the 1992 Women's Health Initiative (WHI), designed to study if hormone replacement in menopause could prevent cardiovascular disease, the average age of the participant was 63 years. Moreover, Premarin® (a mixture of estrogens extracted from the urine of pregnant mares), combined with the synthetic progesterone, medroxyprogesterone, was administered as Prempro®. We now know that it was the wrong age group to study this question. Moreover, oral estrogen, with its first pass through the liver after intestinal absorption, increases the risk of blood clots and stroke. And the synthetic progesterone used may well have contributed to the increase in breast cancer observed in the Prempro® group, since women receiving only Premarin® in that study actually showed a reduction in incidence and deaths from breast cancer.

Most hormones currently provided by compounded pharmacies and pharmaceutical companies are called bioidentical hormones. They are identical in structure and function to your own hormones but are derived from plants. When administered as a patch applied to the lower abdomen once or twice a week, depending on the brand, estradiol is introduced at a low, steady rate through the skin directly into the bloodstream exactly as the ovaries provided estradiol to your body during the reproductive years. There is no first-pass phenomenon as is seen with oral hormones. For women who still have a uterus, progesterone is needed in order to prevent uterine cancer caused by estrogen stimulation.

Today, the benefits of transdermal estradiol during menopause far exceed the risks identified during the Premarin® era. Moreover, initiating hormone replacement earlier in menopause actually decreases cardiovascular and bone risk while benefiting common menopausal symptoms.

Knowledge in the field of menopause medicine is rapidly improving.

Through books, the internet, and care provider contact, educated patients today can have a more sophisticated conversation about this important chapter of their lives. Together, we can make menopause not just tolerable but part of a better you.

⬚⬚

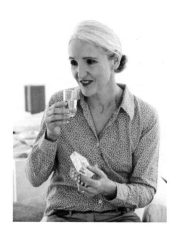

UPDATE ON TIMING OF HORMONE REPLACEMENT THERAPY IN MENOPAUSE

In 1968, Dr. Robert Wilson, a gynecologist in New York City, advocated in his book *Feminine Forever* that all menopausal women should receive hormone replacement therapy (HRT). The outrage of the feminist movement led the National Institutes of Health (NIH) to fund the Women's Health Initiative (WHI) in 1991 to determine if HRT could safely protect women's cardiovascular and bone health. In July 2002, the trial was prematurely canceled due to findings of a statistical increase in both breast cancer and stroke. Based on these findings and the resultant publicity, millions of women stopped their HRT, and doctors stopped prescribing HRT. As a result of this precipitous change, the majority of menopausal women have gone without HRT for more than a decade.

Since the WHI trial, there have been significant improvements in hormone replacement. The WHI utilized only oral conjugated estrogen (Premarin®) alone or combined with medroxyprogesterone acetate (Provera) as Prempro®. Bioidentical estrogen in the form of estradiol and pure micronized progesterone have largely replaced these hormones now, and they are more likely to be given in skin patch, cream, mist, or suppository form as a much safer vehicle to lessen liver and blood clotting effects. The starting age for HRT is now the beginning of menopause (late 40s to early 50s) for the purpose of treating vasomotor symptoms (VMS) with the lowest estrogen dose. The WHI average starting age was 63 years, which generally would not be condoned now.

Currently, duration of treatment of VMS with HRT is also undergoing reevaluation. Older teaching was that VMS for the majority of menopausal women only lasts one to three years. However, in keeping with the experience of most practitioners and their menopausal patients, the recently published Study of Women's Health Across the Nation (SWAN) provides a more protracted picture of VMS. In a group of 3,302 menopausal women from seven US sites who were followed from 1996 to 2013, 1,449 had VMS with a median duration of 7.4 years. Those who experienced VMS as they entered menopause had symptoms lasting longer than 11.8 years (median). Some women have VMS their whole postmenopausal life!

Does treatment of VMS make a difference? Vasomotor symptoms are associated with poorer quality of life, negative moods, and sleep disorders. From subjective symptoms to objective science, recent studies now link VMS to inflammatory and hematologic indicators of increased cardiovascular risk. Women with greater than six days of hot flashes in two weeks exhibit increases in procoagulant/ antifibrinolitic hematologic markers, tissue plasminogen activator (t-PA) antigen, and Factor VII, all of which demonstrate a link between vascular endothelial factors and autonomic neurogenic activity (VMS). Moreover, women with VMS exhibit lower bone mineral density compared to those without VMS. Lower bone density with longer life span portends increased osteoporosis with all of its sequelae in later life. Based on these findings, it is not surprising that VMS have an impact on the economy. Data from over 500,000 Fortune 500 health insurance claims from 1999 to 2011 show that for menopausal women experiencing untreated VMS, there were 57% more indirect productivity days lost (mostly absenteeism) compared to women treated for VMS at an incremental direct yearly cost of $339,599,459 or $770 per person per year.

Proper management of VMS has entered a new era. Based on compounds with improved safety, newer methods of hormone delivery, and awareness of the negative impact and duration of untreated symptoms, HRT has improved the lives of many menopausal women who in the recent past were forced to endure the heat-searing effects of VMS. We can only expect further improvements in our understanding and management of this important women's health issue in the future.

MENOPAUSE TRANSITION

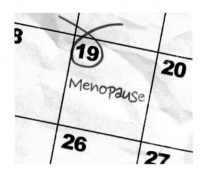

MENOPAUSE OR MENOPAUSE TRANSITION:
WHEN DOES THE BIOLOGY BEGIN?

Does menopause really begin only after a woman experiences her last menstrual period? On average, the age of these women is 51 years. But ask any woman in menopause how she recalls the three to five years before she reached that milestone and most will remember that their menstrual cycles became more erratic and unpredictable. We now know that other biological changes also are beginning to occur.

The official statement of the North American Menopause Society (2012) marks the Menopause transition as a several-year window. It begins with early perimenopause of variable length signaled by fluctuating follicle stimulating hormone (FSH) levels as declining estrogens from the ovaries fail to produce a negative feedback to the brain. A late perimenopause of one to three years is marked by consistently rising FSH levels as estrogen levels fall further, followed by early menopause which lasts for two to six years during which FSH levels stabilize at a high level into late menopause. But what has this to do with the many symptoms that women experience in this chapter of their lives? For those answers, we must examine the critical relationship that exists between estrogen and inflammation.

In the reproductive years, estradiol, 95% of which is produced by the ovaries, functions as the most powerful estrogen. It was always respected for its role in pregnancy and menstrual cycling. Yet, more recently, scientists have shown that during those years estradiol also serves to suppress the response to critical inflammatory proteins such as interleukin 1 (IL-1), interleukin 6 (IL-6) and tumor necrosis factor alpha (TNF a), which are normally generated by monocytes, macrophages, neutrophils, and other cell populations. These inflammatory proteins, when expressed, are capable of stimulating over 60 other inflammatory proteins that we now recognize attack brain, bone, heart, skin, and blood vessels. The appearance of these inflammatory proteins parallels the fluctuating and then rapidly declining estrogen levels seen in late perimenopause.

Women may recognize this period of their lives only by the onset of irregular menstrual periods. Yet it is during this window of time that estrogen levels fluctuate and even may increase briefly before beginning to decline permanently. It is also a time when some women for the first time begin to experience transient hot flashes, mood disorders, vaginal dryness, or sleep disorders.

From clinical studies, scientists also have shown that during the three to five years leading up to the last menstrual period, visceral fat that surrounds our abdominal organs and coats our blood vessels increases to a greater degree than does subcutaneous fat. These specialized fat cells act as tiny factories to produce a wide range of inflammatory proteins. These changes are accompanied by a rise in blood lipid levels and increases in blood vessel wall thickness. These cardiovascular events, while perhaps not generating the emotional reaction of many of the other perimenopausal symptoms, signal the real risk in menopause, that of a cardiovascular event and even stroke.

As scientists continue to clarify the biology of the menopause transition, they will offer clinicians and their patient's education and novel approaches to accommodate this most natural time in life.

⧠⧠

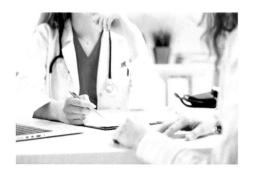

MENOPAUSE TRANSITION: DON'T MISS THIS IMPORTANT PREVENTATIVE HEALTH OPPORTUNITY

Sometime between ages 45 and 55, for many women, gynecologic and related health issues begin to emerge. Menstrual cycles now seem different, mood swings and memory lapses appear, and sleep becomes more chaotic, coupled with warm flushes. And the weight! Why at the mid-section? These irritating acknowledgements belie a more ominous change. During this menopause transition, loosely referred to as "perimenopause," events are unfolding that have an impact on a woman's cardiovascular risk.

The origin of these seemingly unrelated responses falls to the unpredictable decline in estradiol from the ovaries occurring during the 40s and early 50s. Initially produced at high levels during the reproductive years, estradiol's decline as ovaries age is more than simply a change in blood levels. This decline in estradiol eliminates perhaps its most important role, that of a powerful anti-inflammatory hormone. During the reproductive years, estradiol protects the body from damage from inflammatory proteins, called cytokines, normally generated by our visceral fat cells and immune cells that, unheeded, produce many of the irritating menopause symptoms described by women. The decline in the protective anti-inflammatory actions of estradiol can contribute to the development of metabolic syndrome, i.e., abnormal lipid profile, insulin resistance, type 2 diabetes mellitus,

41

and hypertension. Unfortunately, there is no other significant bodily source of estradiol to compensate for this ovarian aging.

While obesity would seem to be the instigator of these changes, this process actually may begin in the brain. Within the hypothalamus, a small group of neurons serve several governing functions. During the reproductive years, they control reproduction by activating the hypothalamic-pituitary-ovarian axis to produce estradiol, maintain the stability of our heat control center in our brain, and help regulate our intestinal proteins. As the ovaries age, declining levels of estradiol result in changes in our ability to reproduce, regulate our body heat, and control our food intake. Ovulation ceases, hot flashes begin to occur, and there is a change in our intestinal proteins as well. The result is an increase in visceral fat and, with that, the emergence of insulin resistance. Therein lies a major contributor to the increased cardiovascular risk in the menopause transition.

Insulin, under normal conditions, utilizes the PI 3 kinase pathway to break down fat (lipolysis) and oxidize glucose for cellular metabolism. But it also is critical for amino acid transport, cell proliferation, and generation of nitric oxide, a potent vasodilator that protects vascular endothelial cells. Visceral fat inhibits the PI 3 kinase pathway, leading to excessive insulin production (hyperinsulinemia). Yet, absent its normal metabolic feedback pathway, increased insulin compensates by utilizing an alternative pathway, the ERK MAP kinase pathway, which offers no metabolic benefit, but which reduces nitric oxide production and, by other proinflammatory steps, increases the risk of atherosclerotic damage. But, could there be another explanation for the inflammation of menopause that produces cardiovascular risk?

New research suggests that the loss of anti-inflammatory properties which parallels the fall of estradiol also could impact a more remote region of the body, one's intestinal bacteria called the intestinal microbita. Our intestine contains about 1014 microbes representing over 1,000 different species, yet four families of bacteria normally dominate. Microbes on the mucosal surface influence our immune system, while those on the luminal surface are important for energy and metabolism. Alterations in our bowel bacteria, however, have been linked to such inflammatory conditions as rheumatoid arthritis, inflammatory bowel disease, and systemic lupus erythematosus. Increased cardiovascular risk results from the fact that certain intestinal bacteria can release lipopolysaccharides (LPS) from their cell walls that, along with increased free fatty acids, stimulate adipose inflammation and insulin resistance.

The literature is quickly becoming filled with studies demonstrating the cardiovascular risks of the menopause transition. Irrespective of the theory of causation, a strategy for reducing these risks must address 1. a diet emphasizing the fundamentals of the Mediterranean diet, eliminating most carbohydrates (which accelerate our hunger), adding omega 3 fatty acids (which curb our appetite), nuts and grains (for protein); and 2. daily exercise (which helps shift fat to muscle).

It appears that Mother Nature never planned for us to live for many more years after our reproductive years. The menopause transition and the symptoms for which women seek care provide physicians and scientists an opportunity to help women improve how well they live that next large chapter in their lives. Important lifestyle changes, including diet and exercise, as well as counseling, can have a huge impact on newly menopausal women. Based on the current understanding of this important window into menopause, they, and we, now have just such an opportunity.

HOT FLASHES

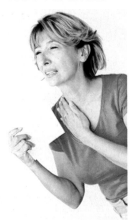

WHAT DO WE KNOW ABOUT HOT FLASHES IN MENOPAUSE?

It is 3 am, and while in bed, you are awakened by a sudden burst of heat in your face, neck, and arms that forces you, now drenched in sweat, to throw off the covers, only then to chill. With up to 75% of women experiencing this phenomenon during the menopause transition and 10% for a lifetime, what do we know about the biology of hot flashes?

Hot flashes are initiated by enhanced sympathetic activity within the brain in association with reduced ovarian estrogen production. Yet, the occurrence of hot flashes correlates poorly with measured levels of plasma, urinary or vaginal estrogen. Hot flashes, however, are linked to elevated baseline plasma levels of norepinephrine metabolites in symptomatic women, which increase further during a hot flash. Estrogen's actions in the brain during ovulation to reduce the response of sympathetic receptors may explain why, during estrogen withdrawal, enhanced sympathetic activity occurs. But how does this explain the clinical picture of hot flashes?

Scientists have found that, during the reproductive years, a woman can adjust to a change in her environment of about 0.4 degrees C without stimulating the hypothalamus, the thermoregulatory part of her brain. Entering a warm room, smoking a cigarette, or having spicy food; these events do not seem to stimulate a central sympathetic response. This is referred to as the "thermoneutral zone." Yet, in the menopausal years, coincidental with a drop in estrogen levels, the thermoneutral zone disappears. This change has been reproduced in the animal model where administering norepinephrine into the blood stream also narrows the thermoneutral zone. Any small rise in temperature then triggers the hypothalamus into action with the goal to lower the body's temperature. As a result, one's heart rate increases to direct capillary blood flow to the skin and moisture is released through the sweat glands, both intended to reduce one's body temperature. Then a brief drop in body temperature occurs, the chill factor.

Treatments using cognitive behavioral therapy, or mind-body interventions such as yoga, hypnosis, or acupuncture, effectively reduce one's response to hot flashes but have little or no effect on frequency. Nonetheless, these approaches have been shown to improve one's response to stress, sleep disorders, and depression. Moreover, dietary modification and weight loss have been shown to reduce vasomotor symptoms.

Estrogen is the gold standard medication for treating hot flashes, usually reducing their incidence and severity. The effectiveness of other treatments must be judged against their placebo effect, the lessening of symptoms based on the woman's expectation that the treatment will work. For those who cannot take systemic estrogens, treatment with clonidine; the Selective Serotonin Reuptake inhibitors (SSRIs) fluoxetine, paroxetine, or sertraline; or the anticonvulsant gabapentin, have all been reported to reduce hot flashes from 20% to 50% of women tested.

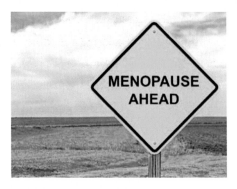

HOT FLASH CONNECTION TO PUBERTY

Puberty is a dynamic process that occurs as young women emerge into their reproductive lives. The pre-pubertal process begins in the hypothalamus. There, cells called gonadotrophin-releasing hormone neurons secrete gonadotrophin-releasing hormone (GnRH). GnRH in turn enters the portal system in pulses to stimulate the pituitary to produce luteinizing hormone (LH) and follicle-stimulating hormone (FSH), both of which act on the maturing ovary to initiate the production of estrogens and androgens and then progesterone once ovulation occurs. Once produced, rising levels of estrogen communicate back to the hypothalamus to slow the process. But how does estrogen control this feedback process since there are no estrogen receptors on the GnRH neurons? And what does this have to do with menopausal hot flashes?

Scientists have identified a small group of KNDy neurons nestled in the hypothalamus called kisspeptin, neurokinin B and dynorphin (KNDy, pronounced "candy"). Kisspeptin and neurokinin B, stimulatory neurons, and Dynorphin, an inhibitory neuron, act as switches to turn on/off the pre-pubertal GnRH neurons and later, hormone production during the menstrual cycle. KNDy neurons are present in the newborn but are inactive. Their emergence to initiate puberty results from the removal of a series of repressor genes that have kept KNDy neurons quiet since birth. Once these repressor genes are inactivated, the KNDy neurons initiate their stimulation of the GnRH neurons and the whole pubertal process begins.

The role of these stimulatory or inhibitory KNDy neurons in controlling the hot flashes of menopause reflects their location in the brain. KNDy neurons are nestled adjacent to and send fibers into a cluster of neurons in our hypothalamus responsible for thermal regulation. During reproductive life, when estradiol from the ovaries is plentiful, the female body only tolerates about a half of a degree of variation in body temperature without activating compensation within the central nervous system (CNS). This explains why spicy foods, a glass of wine, or mild and brief temperature changes in the environment do not elicit a major response.

Age and the decline in estrogen levels change these dynamics. During menopause the half degree of thermal tolerance is lost; thus, small changes in our body temperature, so slight that one may not even perceive the change, send a powerful signal to the CNS to dilate blood vessels and stimulate sweat glands to release moisture, both of which are mechanisms to lower temperature.

The role of KNDy neurons becomes critical to this process. Hot flashes are characterized by increased GnRH and increased pulsatile secretion of LH. By measuring dilation of blood vessels in the female hairless mouse tail as a model for studying hot flashes, scientists have found that removing the ovaries (and therefore eliminating estradiol from the system) stimulates GnRH and subsequent LH release, both characteristic of hot flashes, thus promoting vasodilation. Ablating the KNDy neurons, including their projections to the hypothalamus, eliminates the LH surge and eliminates vasodilation. Neuroanatomic analyses from premenopausal and postmenopausal women who died from unrelated causes support this theory. A critical reduction in the inhibitory dynorphin neurons in postmenopausal women was noted, thus allowing kisspeptin and neurokinin B to function unopposed leading to GnRH and LH release and less thermal tolerance.

Hot flashes, once thought to be a unique event in menopause, are now understood to be part of a much more robust biology that is related to adolescence. Armed with this knowledge of the function of the KNDy neurons, scientists can look for new approaches to hot flashes.

⏸

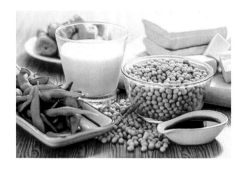

IS SOY A REMEDY FOR HOT FLASHES?

Essentially, everyone has heard the term "soy" as in edamame soy beans, soy flour, tempeh, tofu, soy milk, or soy sauce; a multibillion dollar industry. Why so popular? Perhaps, it is because many of our currently available commercial hormone preparations originate from soy. And for women of Asian descent raised on a diet rich in soy, the rates of hot flashes and breast cancer are reduced significantly compared to those of North American women.

The biology of soy is complex and only partially understood. Soy is a plant protein containing phytoestrogens (hormones derived from plants) called isoflavones , which have an estrogen-like structure that binds weakly to estrogen receptors. Soy isoflavons have been described as either stimulating or blocking estrogen responses. If soy isoflavones attach to estrogen receptors not normally involved in the body's hormone function, their actions are considered stimulating. If they occupy important receptors that need the body's own estrogens, they act as a blocking agent.

Soy isoflavones are made up of genistein, diadzedin, and other lesser soy metabolites. Whole soy beans have equal amounts of genistein and diadzedin, while the soybean germ has four times as much diadzedin as genistein. All commercial soy isoflavones are attached to sugar molecules, which may make up as much as 50%

of the isoflavone. During consumption, sugar is removed in the intestine, resulting in a metabolically active aglycone (without sugar) isoflavone. The intestinal bacteria then convert most of the aglycone into the isoflavone metabolites equol, a daidzedin metabolite, which can be measured in the urine, and p-ethylphenol, both of which are then absorbed into the blood stream. Equol, the more important of the two, has two forms, S(-) equol, believed to be the active form, and R(+) Equol. In one six-month clinical trial in which women were administered a placebo or soy isoflavones, those that demonstrated equol in their urine reported a significantly reduced number of hot flashes, less excessive sweating, fewer palpitations, and less weakness and limb parasthesias when compared with those who received a placebo or when compared with isoflavone-treated women who did not produce equol. Unfortunately, only 20% to 30% of Western women produce S(-) equol, as compared to 50% to 60% of Asian women, which may explain the differences in hot flashes and breast cancer risk between the two populations.

The future direction of soy research is predicated on understanding better how soy interacts with individual estrogen receptors and the inflammatory proteins of menopause. Soy isoflavones are about one third as effective as estrogen in reducing hot flashes. However, prolonged daily soy consumption has been shown to reduce important menopause-related inflammatory proteins.

The role of soy biology is important, and it will be the scientists, working with clinicians, who ultimately define its usefulness in menopause management.

OBESITY AND CARDIOVASCULAR RISK

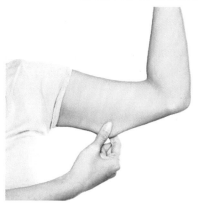

IS ALL BODY FAT THE SAME?

Considerable progress has been made in understanding the role of obesity in healthcare. The old concept was that all fat was bad; that it was associated with hypertension and diabetes. Yet, some more recent studies report that certain overweight or obese individuals actually do not demonstrate these health risks. Now we are beginning to understand why.

Body fat can be divided into subcutaneous fat and visceral fat. Subcutaneous fat is the fat that is deposited on our hips, buttock, arms, and belly. This fat does not seem to carry the health risks of visceral fat. Visceral fat, on the other hand, is fat that is deposited around our abdominal organs but also around our heart. Unlike subcutaneous fat, visceral fat cells are capable of generating many of the inflammatory proteins that attack our blood vessels and our heart. They also may play an important role in many other perimenopausal or menopausal conditions, such as memory loss, mood disorders, hot flashes, bone loss, and skin changes.

How do clinical scientists know where these fat deposits reside in our body? The gold standard for assessing body fat is derived from studies using magnetic resonance imaging (MRI) or computerized tomography (CT scan). A close parallel has been found between these sophisticated and expensive methods and measuring hip or hip-to-waist measurements. Recently, ultrasound measurements of the distance from the back of the abdominal wall to the spine (or to the aorta in a modified protocol) has proved as effective as MRI or CT Scan for finding a correlation between these measurements and serum lipid determinations.

But how does the biology support the imaging? Using animal models, investigators have sampled subcutaneous fat and visceral fat and have demonstrated in the laboratory that only visceral fat cells generate the inflammatory proteins interleukin-1, interleukin 6, and Tumor Necrosis Factor alpha (TNF alpha), the same proteins that have been linked to most menopausal symptoms.

Do both types of fat increase in a similar way throughout life? No. Subcutaneous fat increases gradually as a product of aging and reduced activity. Visceral fat, on the other hand, rapidly increases in the three to five years prior to onset of menopause. Accompanying that increase in visceral fat are increases in carotid artery wall thickness and alterations in one's lipid profile.

Is there any good news? Yes. When begun in earnest, exercise associated with diet control reduces visceral fat more quickly than subcutaneous fat.

⬚⬚

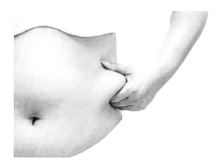

WHAT HAS ESTROGEN GOT TO DO WITH BELLY FAT?

No one likes belly fat since it usually is a reflection of overall elevated weight. Phrases like "pot belly," "beer belly," or "appleshaped" impact both our self-image and our relationship to others. While genetics definitely has some effect, evolutionary forces are also at work here. Does the pattern of fat deposition suggest additional health risks? Why do women seem to preferentially gain belly fat during menopause?

Obesity is indeed a byproduct of evolution. The Paleolithic diet needed to support foraging and chasing down wild animals for food (and thus survival) consisted of red meat, fish, nuts, fruits, and vegetables. This diet was low in carbohydrates and high in proteins and micronutrients. In addition, the Paleolithic lifestyle was very active. In contrast, the industrial revolution brought with it cheap transportation, time-saving machines, high-glycemic prepackaged foods, and resultant obesity.

Unfortunately, fat deposition patterns can reflect health risks. Our superficial fat carries little health risk apart from impacting our psyche and our joints. It is the visceral fat around our internal organs and blood vessels that produces the inflammatory proteins that generate the major health risks of obesity. These intraabdominal fat cells with a direct effect on the liver are linked to the metabolic syndrome with a higher risk of diabetes mellitus, elevated cholesterol and lipids, and resultant cardiovascular disease.

Fat deposition changes with age and sex. Weight gain and fat deposition are similar in boys and girls until puberty. As adolescents, with boys having higher testosterone levels and girls having higher estrogen levels, girls begin to have a higher percentage of body fat. Testosterone causes higher muscle-to-fat ratios as well as its more masculinizing effects. Estrogen causes a typical female fat distribution pattern in breasts, buttocks, and thighs, as well as its more feminizing effects. During the reproductive years, women get additional fat deposition in the pelvis, buttocks, thighs, and breasts to provide an energy source for eventual pregnancy and lactation.

Paradoxically, in menopause, a woman's estrogen levels are inversely related to her weight. In a study of newly menopausal healthy women over a four-year period, women showed an increase in weight and body fat (primarily as visceral adipose tissue), which coincided with a drop in estradiol levels and a decrease in physical activity and energy expenditure. In the laboratory, when female mice were surgically thrust into menopause by removing their ovaries, only those mice treated with estrogen maintained their weight while those deprived of estrogen rapidly gained weight. Why would this be? Studies have shown that estrogen incorporates crucial elements into the DNA responsible for weight control. The absence of both estrogen and these crucial elements leads to progressive obesity.

So, along with hot flashes, irregular menses, irritability, and depression in the menopausal transition, women have to deal with a tendency to weight gain and visceral body fat deposition that can affect their long-term health. The best way to deal with this is still dietary adjustment and increased activity levels.

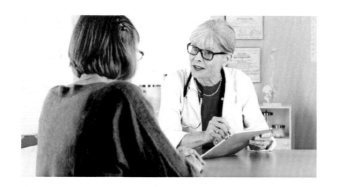

METABOLIC SYNDROME AND THE ROLE OF ESTROGEN

Metabolic syndrome represents a cluster of adverse biologic events characterized by alterations in lipids, elevated blood sugar, and increased cardiovascular risk. According to the National Cholesterol Education Program's Adult Treatment Panel 111 Report, metabolic syndrome may be diagnosed when three of the following criteria are present: waist circumference greater than 88 cm, HDL-C less than 50 mg/dL, triglycerides greater than 150 mg/dL, blood pressure above 130/85 mmHg, or fasting blood sugar over 110 mg/dL. The greatest health risk of metabolic syndrome is cardiovascular disease, but this risk also is age related. Sixty percent of postmenopausal women are affected by metabolic syndrome, whereas only 22% of the general population meet these criteria. These differences in prevalence underscore the dramatic physiologic changes that occur as a woman enters menopause.

Menopause is defined as one year without menses. The menopause transition now is formally defined as the three-to-five-year period leading up to this new stage of life. This transition often is recognized by women with the onset of irregular menses and vasomotor symptoms. Often, it is characterized by increased fat depositions, especially in the intra-abdominal area (visceral fat) with little change in muscle mass. Visceral fat cells with direct access to portal blood entering the liver are a significant source of many of the inflammatory proteins felt to be responsible for cardiovascular heart disease. The appearance of these inflammatory proteins results from fluctuations and then the natural decline of ovarian estradiol, a hormone that in the pre-menopause provides anti-inflammatory protection.

Visceral obesity also correlates closely with an increase in insulin resistance leading to elevated insulin levels, abnormal glucose metabolism, and a reduction in fat breakdown. Insulin, acting through its receptors to stimulate insulin-like growth factor-2 (IGF2), is critical for normal glucose metabolism. It transports glucose from the blood into the cells and allows fat to be broken down. Yet, insulin receptors are under hormonal control since estradiol improves insulin sensitivity and glucose metabolism while reducing body fat. Obesity, coupled with insulin resistance, results in over expression of insulin receptors, lower than normal levels of IGF-2, and production of a second growth factor, insulin-like growth factor -1 (IGF-1), which causes a pathologic process that destabilizes glucose metabolism in insulin-sensitive tissue.

Visceral fat also has a direct effect to increase appetite and reduce energy expenditure. Premenopausal estradiol maintains a balance of intestinal peptides that signal the brain when a person has eaten enough. In these women, appetite is controlled by increased adiponectin and ghrelin and decreased resistin and leptin. Yet, in obese women with metabolic syndrome and insulin resistance, adiponectin (important for cardiovascular protection) is decreased, and leptin and resistin are increased. How do we know estradiol is involved? Transdermal estradiol supplementation in these women reverses these changes. Moreover, in clinical studies, energy expenditure in obese women with metabolic syndrome is reduced but improves once transdermal estradiol supplementation is instituted.

It is not surprising that obesity, especially in the menopause transition, appears to be the primary clinical target for reducing the risk from the metabolic syndrome. Daily exercise and diet management to reduce fat, especially visceral fat, is central to this effort. Moreover, hormone supplementation with transdermal estradiol capitalizes on the effect of estradiol to increase insulin sensitivity, reduce abdominal fat, and rebalance intestinal satiety peptides.

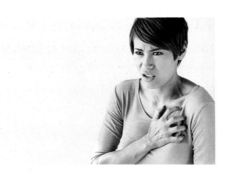

MATTERS OF THE HEART

As they age, men and women differ in one of the most significant aspects of life—matters of the heart. No, not the emotional side of the heart, but the physical side of heart health. For many women in the United States, menopause presents a range of recognized symptoms including hot flashes, weight gain, mood swings, and vaginal pain and dryness on intercourse. These changes can affect quality of life but seldom are lethal. More insidious are risks of breast cancer and osteoporosis. Yet, heart disease is THE leading cause of death among women in America.

Common early symptoms of heart disease are more subtle for women than those for men. The classic male presentation is pain along the left arm and jaw coupled with tightening and pain in the chest. These recognized symptoms are likely to initiate an emergency room visit, immediate cardiac evaluation, and likelihood of coronary angiography with possible stent placement or coronary bypass surgery. For women, the early symptom of heart disease most frequently seen is unusual fatigue, but some women experience sleep disorders, shortness of breath, indigestion, anxiety, and even rarely, chest discomfort. These complaints are dismissed easily as reflecting the stresses of everyday life. The vague nature of these complaints helps explain the reduced use of cardiac evaluations when women present with these symptoms. Healthcare providers need to have a high index of suspicion when evaluating women with fatigue and/or these other symptoms to consider cardiac disease after ruling out anemia, thyroid disease, depression, and anxiety along with other more rare disorders.

The biologic differences in heart disease between men and women help explain the contrasting symptoms. For men, a heart attack is preceded by a series of biologic events in which oxidized cholesterol damages the endothelial cells lining the coronary arteries. These damaged cells draw immune cells from the blood into the coronary artery wall where they help develop into a space occupying plaque which can lead to compromised blood flow. If and when this plaque finally ruptures, a thrombus (clot) blocks the artery leading to cardiac muscle damage and possible death. For women, presumably due to the unique hormonal environment, only tiny lipid plaques form and are distributed throughout the smaller coronary blood vessels, which probably explains the more subtle symptoms of women's heart disease.

Both family history and lifestyle contribute to defining a person's risk of heart disease. A strong family history increases risk, and that component of heart health is non-preventable. In contrast, we can control many lifestyle factors. Smoking is the leading modifiable risk factor linked to heart disease, yet obesity is not far behind. Estimates are that two-thirds of menopausal women are overweight or obese, and with obesity comes increased insulin resistance and a heightened risk of diabetes. While our subcutaneous (SQ) fat is esthetically unpleasant, it is the visceral fat (around our organs and inside our abdomen) that produces many of the inflammatory proteins linked to heart disease. Moreover, visceral fat cells also exist as a thin fat layer lying directly on our blood vessels, thereby giving their inflammatory proteins direct access to our circulation. Fortunately, studies have shown that weight loss efforts (diet and exercise) can reduce both SQ and visceral fat.

While women's heart health may seem complex, we have made significant advances in educating both providers and women regarding identifying at-risk groups and early diagnosis of heart disease. There is now more emphasis than ever on preventive and predictive measures in women's heart health with the hope of decreasing heart disease as the leading killer of women.

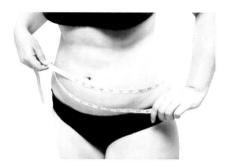

MENOPAUSE, METABOLISM, AND VISCERAL FAT ACCUMULATION

Our bodies, anthropologically, function solely to reproduce in order to preserve our species. But reproduction requires adequate metabolic energy. Witness the increase in body fat as one enters puberty or the negative effect on fertility for patients with anorexia nervosa, for those engaging in strenuous exercise, or those subjected to famine and starvation. Yet, as our ability to reproduce ceases at the other end of the age spectrum, we experience a reduction in metabolism, redistribution of fat to our abdominal area and, thus, the cardiovascular and diabetic risks of metabolic syndrome. The key to these interactions resides in our hypothalamus where reproduction and metabolism are controlled.

Reproduction is initiated by three small groups of neurons in our hypothalamus called the KNDy neurons (kisspeptin, neurokinin B, and dynorphin) pronounced "candy." In the adolescent child, as puberty approaches, suppressor genes that have kept these neurons quiet since birth lose their inhibitory effect. These KNDy neurons, with direct connections to our gonadotrophin-releasing hormone (GnRH) neurons, stimulate the release of gonadotrophin-releasing hormone (GnRH). GnRH, in turn, activates the pituitary to produce pulsatile luteinizing hormone (LH) and follicle-stimulating hormone (FSH), both of which stimulate the ovaries to begin to produce cyclic estrogen and progesterone, and the reproductive cycle begins.

These KNDy neurons, however, also play an important role in regulating metabolism by responding to feedback from peripheral hormones that are responsible for appetite and nutritional absorption. While more complex than stated here, in brief, leptin released from our white fat and insulin from our pancreas decrease our appetite and tell us to eat less. In contrast, ghrelin, from our gut, increases our appetite, usually causing us to eat more.

Evidence that our metabolism and reproductive function interact is demonstrated by the fact that caloric restriction leading to ghrelin secretion reduces pulsatile GnRH release from the gonadotrophin-releasing neurons, thereby impairing ovulation. Although metabolism and reproduction must work collaboratively, reproductive processes do not respond directly to metabolic cues. For example, GnRH neurons have no leptin or ghrelin receptors, and KNDy neurons have no ghrelin receptors. The higher order control of metabolism to support reproduction is believed to reside at the arcuate nucleus in the hypothalamus, which has access to circulating molecules outside the blood-brain barrier. It also has receptors for leptin, insulin, and ghrelin, and contains regulators of the KNDy and GnRH neurons.

Connecting the dots, however, has left us with one question: "Why does visceral fat form in the months or years leading into menopause?"

The initiating factor may be fluctuation and then loss of ovarian estradiol with its anti-inflammatory properties in the menopause transition, thus altering the immune characteristics of our intestinal bacteria and their control over nutritional absorption. Falling estradiol levels also produce alterations in KNDy neurons (now believed to be the origin of hot flashes) and could facilitate changes in how we metabolize our food. Evidence supporting this theory is found in breast cancer patients treated with aromatase inhibitors who have lowered estrogen levels and both an increasing incidence of hot flashes and increasing abdominal obesity. A contrasting theory, supported by animal and clinical studies, indicates an association between higher androgen levels and visceral fat accumulation. Perhaps both low estrogen and relatively elevated androgen levels contribute to the development of metabolic syndrome phenotype in genetically predisposed perimenopausal women. Other hormones, like thyroid hormone and cortisol, obviously have some role in this process as well.

Visceral fat cells, although only a small component of our overall body fat, accumulate non-esterified free fatty acids faster than subcutaneous fat cells. These visceral fat cells deliver free fatty acids (FFA) via the portal vein directly to our liver, thus contributing a higher proportion of overall hepatic FFA in individuals with greater visceral fat. The results are an increase in very low density lipoproteins (VLDL) and insulin resistance, hallmarks of type 2 diabetes and increased cardiovascular risk.

The biologies of reproduction and of metabolism, once thought of as silos, now seem more integrated. This observation raises new possibilities for novel treatments to prevent metabolic syndrome.

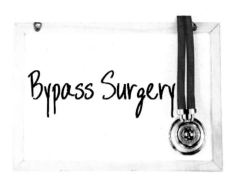

IMPACT OF VARIOUS BARIATRIC PROCEDURES
IN TREATING DIABETES IN MENOPAUSE

Weight control challenges many women entering menopause. For some, weight gain is only an assault on their personal image. For others, however, their abdominal obesity, more so than their total weight gain, significantly increases their risk for type 2 diabetes mellitus and heart disease. Diet and exercise have been the tools for managing weight gain in the past. While effective for some, a more aggressive approach involving bariatric surgery to limit intestinal absorption has been required for those whose body mass index (BMI) places them in the obese category.

There are a number of types of bariatric surgeries designed to reduce weight. Restrictive procedures such as the laparoscopic adjustable gastric banding (LAGB) and vertical banded gastroplasty (VBG) reduce the volume of food in the stomach in order to decrease caloric intake and reduce one's appetite. In contrast, malabsorptive procedures like the biliopancreatic diversion (BPD) shorten the small intestine to decrease absorption of nutrients, while combined procedures like the Roux-en-Y gastric bypass (RYGB) restrict the stomach volume and also alter the small intestine to decrease absorption.

Historically, bariatric surgery was credited with reducing one's BMI by restricting caloric intake and, in some patients, improving their diabetes mellitus, an important secondary benefit since nearly 30% of patients undergoing bariatric surgery have type 2 diabetes. More recently, investigators have noted that certain restrictive bariatric procedures result in rapid resolution or improvement in diabetes within days of the operation, long before the blood glucose improvement could be attributed to weight loss alone. It seems that bariatric procedures that alter absorption in the small intestine affect the peptides within the gut that control insulin secretion, a phenomenon that is not seen following restrictive procedures.

The epithelium of our intestinal tract contains specialized K and L cells (named before their functions were understood) that secrete critical peptides to communicate to our pancreas how to respond to the stimulatory effects of glucose. Glucagon-like peptide-1 (GLP-1) from the L cells of the distal ileum stimulates the pancreatic islets to increase glucose-dependent insulin secretion, slow gastric emptying to control postprandial glycemia, and increase satiety (a sense of fullness). Glucose-dependent insulinotropic peptide (GIP) from the K cells of the proximal gut responds to carbohydrates and fats. Peptide YY (PYY), secreted by L cells of the distal intestine, increases satiety and delays gastric emptying. Ghrelin from the gastric fundus and small intestine regulates appetite in the hypothalamus through increased blood levels before meals and decreased levels after meals.

Two current theories exist to explain this bariatric-diabetic phenomenon. In the "lower intestinal hypothesis" by Cummings (2007), rapid delivery of nutrients to the distal bowel improves glucose metabolism by increasing secretion of GLP-1 and other appetite suppressive gut peptides. The "foregut exclusion theory" of Rubino (2008) instead suggests that bypassing the duodenum and proximal jejunum blocks the secretion of a "signal" that promotes insulin resistance.

While the physiology of this remarkable link between certain bariatric procedures and the rapid improvement in type 2 diabetes mellitus remains to be resolved, the observation itself has made investigators in diabetes management go back to the drawing board to rethink old theories and to construct new approaches to care.

BONE HEALTH

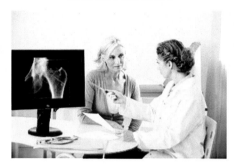

BONE HEALTH: WHAT'S MENOPAUSE GOT TO DO WITH IT?

You may be unaware that your bones are engaging in a balanced, continuous process of remodeling; laying down new bone while eliminating old bone. So why is this process jeopardized in menopause?

Bone is produced by osteoblasts. These cells lay down a material called osteoid, composed of a collagen in a lattice frame, and fill it in with inorganic material called hydroxyapatite, a complex molecule of calcium and phosphate written as $Ca_{10}(PO_4)_6(OH)_2$. Hydroxyapatite gives bone its strength and resiliency, and since it contains 99% of the body's calcium, it serves as the main reservoir when calcium is needed for other bodily processes.

Bone is broken down by osteoclasts, which are derived from stem cells in the blood. Osteoclasts are activated by a group of inflammatory cytokines that stimulate osteoclast activity. When osteoclasts attach to bone matrix, their edges release acid and other substances to dissolve hydroxyapatite, thus releasing calcium, other minerals, and protein materials into the blood and then urine.

Bone turnover is regulated by several factors. Hydroxyapatite requires the availability of calcium which is regulated by vitamin D. Vitamin D3 (called calciferol) is synthetized in the skin by ultraviolet B light. Vitamin

D2 is produced by dietary plants. Both are converted in the liver to 1,25 dihydroxy vitamin D, which controls calcium absorption in the small intestine. Parathyroid hormone (PTH) has little effect on intestinal calcium absorption but stimulates osteoblast activity and promotes calcium reabsorption in the kidney.

Bone strength changes over the lifetime. Peak bone strength occurs between the ages of 20 to 30. During menopause, bone loss accelerates in the three years before and the three years after the final menstrual period at a rate of 2% per year, then slows to 1% a year afterward.

Bone health is measured by Bone Mineral Density (BMD), determined by Dual Energy X-Ray Absorptiometry (DXA Scan). By this technique, two X-ray beams of different energy are aimed at bone. The results, presented as a T Score, are compared to that of the average race-matched young normal female. Measurements of -1 to -2.5 Standard Deviations (SD) below peak normal values of the lumbar spine, or femur neck (hip) reflect low bone density (osteopenia) and -2.5 SD or greater reflect significant bone loss (osteoporosis). For white women over 50 years, 13% to 18% have osteoporosis of the hip, and 30% to 50% have osteopenia. By age 80, over 50% are likely to exhibit osteoporosis, making hip fractures, with a 25% mortality rate in the first year, a serious risk.

Age, a family history of osteoporosis, smoking, malnutrition, low estrogen levels, and chronic disease are all risk factors for bone loss. Because natural estradiol inhibits cytokine-induced osteoclast activity, the expected decline of estradiol in menopause contributes to the risk of osteoporosis. Current daily recommendations for menopausal women who are not on estrogen therapy are 800 IU of vitamin D and calcium obtained from the diet. Other preventive measures include weight-bearing exercises, fall prevention strategies like Tai Chi, and hormone therapy that includes estrogen. All can decrease a woman's risk of bone loss.

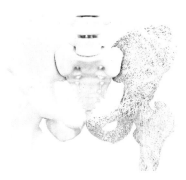

THE VALUE OF MONITORING BONE HEALTH WITH AGING

Our ability to monitor and, hopefully, improve aging bone health is the product of modern technology and a renewed focus on preventative medicine. Terms such as "DXA (previously dexa) scans," and "T-scores" populate our discussion of aging and the prevention of falls. But the negative impact of a hip fracture cannot be overestimated. In one study of 428 consecutive hip fracture patients followed for up to 3.7 years, the risk of mortality was three-fold higher than that of the general population over 65 years of age. In another series of 758 hip fracture patients over 60 years of age, 21% died in the first year, despite being co-managed by orthopedic surgeons and geriatricians. Why are certain bones in our body at greater risk of fracture than others, and how do we monitor and affect that risk?

Healthy bones are a result of a continuous process, from birth until death, of modeling and remodeling to adapt to normal biomechanical and hormonal forces and additionally to repair damaged bone. Bones are made up of 50% to 70% mineral (primarily hydroxyapatite for mechanical rigidity and strength), 24% to 40% organic matrix (primarily collagen 1 for elasticity), 5% to 10% water, and less than 3% lipids. Long bones (for example the humerus, radius, ulnar, and femur) have a hollow shaft made of hard, cortical (compact) bone for support and movement, which encloses the marrow space and trabecular (cancellous or spongy) bone on the ends. Trabecular bone and marrow function to maintain hematopoiesis, mineral homeostasis, and a reservoir for growth factors. Trabecular bone, which is a honey-combed lattice of trabecular plates and rods, also is found in the flat bones of the skull, ribs, vertebrae, and pelvis. The human skeleton consists of 80% cortical bone and 20% trabecular bone, but this relationship differs by site. The ratio of cortical to trabecular bone in the vertebrae is 25/75, while in the femoral head it is 50/50.

Modeling of new bone begins *in utero* as bone-building cells called osteoblasts manufacture matrix, which is made up mostly of collagen into which calcium compounds, mostly calcium phosphate, are deposited. These cells then become osteocytes, which are surrounded by calcified matrix and serve to monitor mechanical stresses and, through signaling molecules, coordinate the balance between bone production by osteoblasts and bone breakdown by osteoclasts. Throughout life, as bone requires remodeling or repair, new osteoblasts develop from stem cells that come from the dense vascular connective tissue that lines the outer aspect of compact bone (periosteum) and the inner surface lining of the bone's marrow cavity (endosteum). Resorption of "old" bone involves a different cell type called osteoclasts. Osteoclasts are large, multinucleated cells derived from the monocyte-macrophage cell line that have the ability to lower the pH in bone, which mobilizes bone material, thus allowing it to be removed and excreted. In a single year, approximately 20% of bone tissue is replaced.

The challenge in managing bone health is the impact of aging. During menopause, women lose about 1% to 2% of bone per year, mostly in the first couple of years, as bone resorption exceeds bone deposition, linked in part to the decline in estradiol from the ovaries. Other factors besides age that affect the development of osteopenia (mildly reduced bone mass) and osteoporosis (severely reduced bone mass to the point of bone brittleness) are family history, race, nutrition, gender, body weight, medications, and bone structure (frame). Therefore, monitoring the rate of bone loss and, thus, osteoporosis risk in the postmenopausal female has become a major preventative health issue.

Prior to 1987, bone status testing was a plain X-ray of the skeleton, which was poor at determining bone density. Single- and then dual-photon absorptiometry were introduced, focused first on the radius (single) and then on the spine and femur, but both used radioactive isotopes as energy sources. Introduction of dual-energy X-ray eliminated problems with decaying isotopes. Then, in 1987, Hologic® first introduced dual-energy X-ray absorptiometry (DXA), which generated alternate high- and low-energy pulses in a thin beam. Soft tissue absorption was subtracted, leaving values only for bone mineral density (BMD). Although a DXA scan did not determine structural or mechanical strength, its use gained attention in 1990 when reports first appeared that bisphosphonates can slow the process of bone resorption. Fracture risk as a T score from DXA measurements was established as the negative or left shift of a bell curve distribution of values from adults with a fracture history compared to that of healthy young adults without fractures. The Study of Osteoporotic Fractures, a ten-year study of 9,704 white women begun in the United States in the 1980s, found that a T score from the femoral head of -2.5 standard deviations or worse as compared to a normal T score of 0 presented the greatest risk for a subsequent hip fracture.

In 2008, using a meta-analysis of 12 independent studies, the World Health Organization expanded the value of the DXA scan and developed the Fracture Risk Assessment Tool or FRAX score. By using the T score from the femoral neck along with age, body mass index, prior fractures after age 50, family history of hip fractures, smoking and alcohol use, corticosteroid use, or history of rheumatoid arthritis, the ten-year risk of a hip fracture or incidental osteoporotic fracture could then be calculated. Fracture Risk Assessment scores that reflect a greater than 3% risk of a hip fracture or a 20% risk of another bone fracture became justification for offering some type of treatment.

Recent tools to assist care providers in monitoring their patients' bone health involve an array of blood and urine bone turnover markers, which reflect the rate of bone resorption. While bone turnover markers are not used to diagnose osteoporosis, they can assist in managing the pharmacologic treatment of patients at increased risk of osteoporotic fractures.

The important role of the DXA scan is strongly supported by the North American Menopause Society, National Osteoporosis Foundation, American College of Preventive Medicine, and the U.S. Preventive Services Task Force who recommend screening of BMD in all post-menopausal women beginning at the age of 65 or sooner if there are co-morbidities.

Time and research observation will tell if the improved diagnosis and treatment of osteopenia and osteoporosis actually improve morbidity and mortality of the aging U.S. population.

〇〇

VAGINAL INFLAMMATION AND INTIMACY

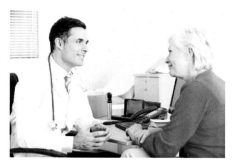

DOCTOR, WHY DOES IT HURT DOWN THERE?

Over 60% of women in menopause complain, often silently, of vaginal dryness and pain during intercourse. As a consequence, they may seek to avoid that level of intimacy, a behavior that can impact negatively on their relationships and, for some, may lead to loneliness and depression. Why?

During the reproductive years, estradiol, produced by the ovaries, is important for health of the vagina, vulva, and lower bladder. Estradiol stimulates nitric oxide, a dilator of blood vessels, to deliver blood with its high water content to the pelvis. This moisture is drawn into the tissues because of the differing concentrations of sodium, potassium, and chloride between blood and vaginal secretions. These ions are important for regulating vaginal lubrication. Estradiol also stimulates the growth of lactobacillis, healthy vaginal bacteria that metabolize glycogen anaerobically to lactic acid in order to maintain the acidity of the vagina at 4 +/-.05, a pH that is hostile to many sexually transmitted infections. Deeper within the tissues, estradiol protects collagen to maintain support and integrity of the vagina, vulva, and bladder.

During menopause, vaginal tissues become dry and shrink. Why? Estradiol's decline results in a reversal of its tissue-protecting effects. Blood vessels decrease in number and size, thus, reducing tissue moisture. Lactobacillis that formerly maintained acidity of the vagina disappear, leading to more alkaline vaginal secretions (normal postmenopausal vaginal pH is 6 to 7.5) and a greater risk of infections. Even the bladder becomes more susceptible to urinary tract infections (UTI). But what makes the vaginal area so vulnerable to these infections? That question takes us to the heart of the problem.

Declining levels of ovarian estradiol lead to chronic inflammation in these tissues, as other cells begin to produce inflammatory proteins that had been chronically suppressed by higher levels of estrogens during the reproductive years. It is the emergence of inflammation in the vaginal area that promotes the repeating infections that women experience. It also explains the pain on intercourse, as vaginal manipulation occurs in the setting of these inflamed tissues.

Systemic hormone replacement may reduce vaginal dryness, but it is not for everyone. Local hormonal therapy in the form of estradiol cream applied to the vagina in small amounts reverses many of these inflammatory-induced effects. However, some women, especially breast cancer survivors, usually are told not to use vaginal estrogen cream due to their risk of increased estrogen blood levels above the normal menopausal range. Yet, due to the estrogen-blocking drugs that many breast cancer survivors take, the problems of vaginal dryness are greater than those of normal menopausal women. Current studies now indicate that androgen creams made of testosterone or dehydroepiandrosterone (DHEA) may offer relief without increasing estrogen blood levels.

Vaginal dryness affects the majority of menopausal women. Fortunately, systemic hormone therapy and local therapies such as estrogen and androgen creams, moisturizers, lubricants, and pH balancers now are available to help.

⌷⌷

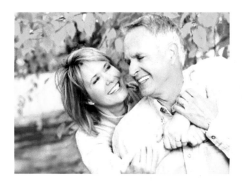

MENOPAUSAL INTIMACY: WHAT'S SEX GOT TO DO WITH IT?

Many women reach menopause and wonder what happened to their sex lives. They feel a decreasing desire for vaginal sex but crave partner intimacy and trust. Sexuality evolves as we age. Intimacy is defined in this context by Webster's Dictionary as a close personal relationship marked by affection and love. It also has been used to denote sexual intercourse. Intimacy in menopause does not necessarily involve sexual intercourse.

Anthropologists tell us that the driving purpose of sexual intercourse is to reproduce the species. Humans are in a rare group of primates in their desire for sexual monogamy. The human desire for sexual intercourse and intimacy continues throughout the lifespan of men and women despite the fact that a woman's ability to reproduce rapidly declines after age 40 and ceases by about age 50.

Hormone blood levels, unfortunately, do not provide a clear picture of why sexual desire and satisfaction change over time for many women. Blood levels of androgens (testosterone, dehydroepiandrosterone sulfate [DHEAS], and androstenedione) decline by two-thirds between age 30 and 70, reaching a lower but stable level during menopause. Unfortunately, women with low libido and those with normal libido can have similar levels. We do know that removal of the ovaries in premenopausal and perimenopausal women can precipitously cause many menopausal symptoms, including decreased desire. Some antidepressant medications also can reduce libido.

A recent AARP survey indicated that over 70% of baby boomers said sex was still important, and 54% were satisfied with their sex life. Yet, 76% indicated that sexual desire had declined in the past 20 years, and by age 75 to 85 only 16% of women and 38% of men were sexually active.

Many emotional changes impact intimacy and sexuality around the time of menopause. Children leaving home, elderly parents becoming more dependent, job stresses, and relationship stresses all can affect sexual feelings. Women, more than men, often need the right "frame of mind" to have increased desire and sexual intimacy. The willingness to become aroused occurs first, followed by sensing the emotion of desire, which can then usually lead to pleasurable sexual intercourse. Emotional and physical obstacles, however, can interfere anywhere along this path. Sexual dysfunction can result from any of the following symptoms: loss of desire, difficulty in arousal or orgasm, occurrence of discomfort or pain, AND personal distress about the problem.

At the end of the day, each woman needs to decide how intimacy and sexual intercourse fit into her life. For many, partner intimacy and sexual satisfaction are not defined by genital function alone but are complemented by friendship, loyalty, history, and trust. Is intimacy reflected by one's sexual activities or, instead, the unanticipated flowers for no reason, the hand that holds yours during the darkest moments of cancer therapy, or the comfort of knowing that the foot touching yours in bed late at night loves you for being you? You choose.

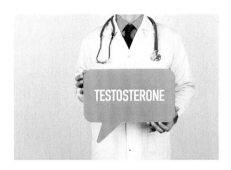

LET'S TALK ABOUT TESTOSTERONE

Some sports figures have abused it. Many men with "low T" have used it. But most women have been refused it. While over 25 testosterone products in the United States are available to men, for women, there are no FDA-approved testosterone products. For vaginal atrophy and pain with intercourse, only estrogen creams or pills are recommended.

The Rio Olympics highlighted the consequences of banned anabolic steroid use when many athletes and a few teams were prevented from competing. Prior Olympic medals are being questioned now in view of modern testing for banned substances. Androgen (anabolic) steroid abuse in sports has been seen in many strength-based sports but is best evidenced in baseball. The steroid era began in 1993, resulting in marked increases in batters' "on-base percentages" and sluggers' hits, which coincided with a sudden rise in the economic value of certain players and major league franchises. The benefits of enhanced strength and athletic performance from these steroids, unfortunately, were offset by increased cardiovascular pathology and cancers of the liver, prostate, and kidney.

In contrast, androgen deficiencies also negatively impact health. "Low T," described by the American Endocrine Society as less than 300 ng/dL in men, does exist and has generated a nearly three-fold increase in prescription testosterone sales. So, what exactly does this hormone do? And why is it important?

Testosterone is produced in several tissues including testes, adrenal cortex, liver, ovaries, and brain from cholesterol-derived dehydroepiandrosterone (DHEA), dehydroepiandrosterone sulfate (DHEA-S), and androstenedione. They are called prehormones, which, when needed, act as inactive reservoirs for subsequent testosterone production. Most testosterone, in turn, also exists in an inactive state, because approximately 98% is bound to proteins called sex hormone binding globulin (SHBG-80%) and albumin (18%). Less than 2% of testosterone is "free" and not bound to a protein, therefore serving as the active hormone.

Testosterone produces its actions in three ways. It directly acts to stimulate protein production in muscle, improves insulin sensitivity, and reduces fat through lipolysis. And it can be converted to dihydrotestosterone (DHT). Dihydrotestosterone blood levels in men are one-tenth those of testosterone, but DHT is five times more active and is responsible for libido, spermatogenesis, muscle development, and bone density. It also can be aromatized to estradiol. Women have only one-tenth of the testosterone blood levels of men, yet their levels of testosterone are approximately ten-fold higher than those of estradiol, making testosterone the most abundant active hormone in the female body. In this complex system in women, androgens influence bone and muscle mass, fat distribution, sexual behavior, libido, thermal control, cognition, visual-spatial skills, and learning.

Age, unfortunately, alters the hormonal picture for both men and women. As men age, androgen levels steadily decline. Since low testosterone is associated with atherosclerotic lipid changes, increased visceral obesity, insulin resistance, and risk of type 2 diabetes mellitus, coronary artery disease becomes a natural consequence of this age-related androgen change. For women, there can be a more abrupt hormonal change, which for some begins even in their late 40s. Ovarian estradiol begins to drop during that period and is often very low in most women by age 52. Women's androgen levels, in contrast, decline over 50% between age 20 and 40, but then remain stable from age 40 to 60 as a result of continued ovarian production. During those few years leading up to and into menopause, many women experience anxiety, depressed mood, decreased libido, and sleep disorders. Is this from the loss of estradiol alone, or is the ratio of estradiol to testosterone critical for women's overall health?

Scientists have focused too long on changes in women's estradiol levels as the sole explanation for their symptoms. Yet, usually the body does not function based on changes in only one hormone but instead functions as an integrated hormonal system. In Europe, transdermal androgen supplementation as a part of integrated hormonal therapy has been used for women during menopause for many years. Vaginal DHEA has been used to treat vaginal atrophy and decreased libido with some success. Testosterone in these low doses has not produced hepatotoxicity, uterine hyperplasia, altered cardiovascular function or coagulation changes, and may even reduce breast cancer risk.

The Food and Drug Administration (FDA) has been concerned with the long-term cardiovascular safety of testosterone therapy in women. As hormone management during menopause gains more acceptance and more long-term data are gathered, it is likely that in the United States and Canada, hormone replacement therapy for some will include the safe addition of testosterone.

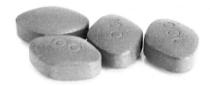

DO WOMEN NEED THEIR OWN "VIAGRA"?

On June 5, 2015, U.S. news headlines proclaimed "FDA Panel Endorses Female Viagra." This was inaccurate, because after two denials, it was only the advisory committee to the Food and Drug Administration (FDA) who voted favorably to recommend that the FDA approve the drug Flibanserin® in August. The FDA wants more information on side effects of the drug, including dizziness, nausea, fatigue, insomnia, and the effects of alcohol. Flibanserin® is touted as a treatment for Hypoactive Sexual Desire Disorder (HSDD) for premenopausal women, which is defined as the persistent lack of sexual fantasies and desire that is distressful to the individual. An estimated 10% of women experience this distress, which is why these headlines caught most people's attention.

Sildenafil (Viagra®) is a performance-enhancing drug for erectile dysfunction, not a form of testosterone. Penile erection results when nitric oxide produces 3'5'cyclic GMP, causing dilation of the blood vessels of the corpus cavernosum of the penis, resulting in an erection. This process is controlled by the enzyme phosphodiesterase (PDE-5), which can inactivate cGMP to impair vasodilation of the penile blood vessels. Sildenafil blocks PDE-5, thus enhancing the effects of cGMP to sustain the erection.

Testosterone therapy has been used off-label as a treatment for HSDD, despite the fact that many studies show no association between androgen therapy and female sexual function. There is no FDA-approved form of testosterone for women. The FDA has remained concerned regarding major (cardiovascular disease and breast cancer) and minor (acne and hair growth) side effects of this drug.

Flibanserin®, in contrast, interacts directly within the complex network of neural hormones in the central nervous system that influence sexual behavior. Sexual arousal and desire are a product of competing influences between the stimulating effects of dopamine and the inhibitory effects of serotonin. Moreover, estrogen and testosterone stimulate dopamine release to enhance sexual desire, while a complex balancing of various serotonin receptors determines the repressive effect of serotonin. Flibanserin® is a serotonin 1A (5 HT1a) receptor agonist, a serotonin 2A (5HT2a) receptor antagonist, and a dopamine D4 receptor partial agonist, meaning the drug has both stimulating and blocking capabilities depending on where in the brain it is functioning.

Results of a number of studies support Flibanserin®'s impact on sexual activity and the neural hormones involved. In rats, increases in norepinephrine (a product of dopamine) and decreases in serotonin were documented in all brain areas associated with sexual behavior. From the FDA Advisory Committee Document (2015) in all three phase 3 human clinical trials of Flibanserin®, women reported improvements in sexuality of 9.4% to 14.6% over placebo-treated women.

Arousal and desire for men and women are as much psychologic as biologic. Basic questions that often dominate any discussion of intimacy in the gynecologist's office are "Do you like yourself? Do you like your partner? Who does the lack of desire or libido bother, you or your partner? And finally, do you want to improve how you feel about your sexuality?" Armed with these answers, the gynecologist is able to navigate toward a more productive discussion and strategy for care.

There is a great deal of interest on the part of pharmaceutical companies to help women with HSDD for obvious market volume reasons. Since sexual desire dysfunction is multifactorial in women, often involving relationship issues and intimacy as well as possible anxiety and/or depression, it is unlikely that one pill will be a simple solution.

◻◻

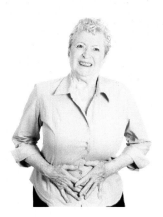

A BRIEF HISTORY OF NONSURGICAL TREATMENTS FOR STRESS URINARY INCONTINENCE

Stress urinary incontinence (SUI), which usually is related to pelvic organ prolapse (POP), is the involuntary leakage of urine with activity or straining such as when a woman is exercising, coughing, or even stepping off a curb. Estimates of 25% to 60% of women experience this over the course of their lifetime, and the numbers increase with increasing age.

A woman's ability to control urinary leakage with exertion requires contraction of the muscles of the external urethral sphincter and physical compression of the proximal urethra which lies within the anterior wall of the vagina. Numerous therapies and nonsurgical procedures have been developed over the years to help correct this problem, including pelvic exercises, pessaries, hormonal treatments, and biofeedback. No single therapy is considered best. The success of any one of these is difficult to measure because of small study numbers and the type and duration of observation. Many times, a combination produces the best outcome.

Physiologic therapy of the pelvic musculature, first championed by Arnold Kegel in the mid-1950s, focused on strengthening the pubococcygeus muscle of the pelvis. This muscle connecting the symphysis pubis to the coccyx sends numerous fibers that insert into the intrinsic musculature of the proximal urethra, middle third of the vagina, and rectum. Today, Kegel exercises are widely used as a first-line treatment promoted by Kegel's early writings describing "complete relief from simple urinary stress incontinence... in a series of over 700 users." A more recent study from the Norwegian Centre for Physiotherapy Research confirmed that patients who performed Kegel exercises significantly improved stress urinary incontinence as compared with those who did not.

Pessaries are synthetic devices that provide artificial mechanical support to the vagina and cervix. They have been used for both POP and SUI. While often promoted as a first-line approach for both, pessary success is often difficult to document because of the many different types of pessaries that can be used and the varying degrees of POP that occur with SUI. Nonetheless, success rates up to 62% for advanced POP have been reported, although less success is achieved if POP is associated with SUI.

Hormone therapy would seem to address menopausal changes in tissues of the vaginal mucosa and lower bladder when ovarian estradiol ceases to be produced. Systemic hormone replacement, however, has failed to correct this problem as demonstrated conclusively in a recent Cochrane review. This conclusion is consistent with other studies in which over 50% of women on systemic hormone replacement, while relieved of generalized menopausal symptoms, continue to experience vaginal atrophy and painful intercourse. Localized vaginal estrogen treatment, in contrast, appears to improve POP and SUI.

Biofeedback, using EMG (electromyography) or surface EMG, is an effective nonsurgical option for moderate SUI with success rates as high as 60%. Combined use of voiding diaries, timed voids, and selective restriction of fluids link behavioral training to physical function. More extensive biofeedback may include the placement of vaginal tension-measuring devices or small electrical sensors on the perineum or in the vagina. These devices are then connected to a computer to display pelvic muscle activity during voluntary pelvic muscle strengthening exercises. Pelvic floor rehabilitation involves strengthening weak pelvic floor muscles (cause of SUI and POP) and controlling spasms in these same muscles (cause of pelvic/perineal pain). Often, a specially trained physical therapist can help guide a patient and develop an effective plan.

The nonsurgical management of stress urinary incontinence is a constantly evolving field involving both old and new innovative treatments. In reality, the use of several of these therapies together often can lead to significant improvement in SUI. Even preoperative pelvic muscle strengthening and re-education with simple behavior modification can improve the results of surgical treatments of SUI, but many times, the nonsurgical treatments alone for some patients can produce enough improvement that surgery is no longer desired.

SKIN AND HAIR

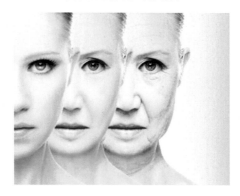

DOES ESTROGEN HELP SKIN AGE BETTER?

Our skin is not only our largest organ but also our protective shield and our most visible self. When Nora Ephron wrote *I Feel Bad about My Neck: And Other Thoughts on Being a Woman* (2008), she was highlighting with humor, but understanding, the challenges women face as they age. And skin becomes a very visible part of that conversation. Why does our skin thin, and what causes wrinkles?

Our skin consists of three important layers. The most superficial layer, the epidermis, contains skin pigmentation, offers protection, and retains moisture. The layer below the epidermis, the dermis, contains hair follicles, nerves, blood vessels, sweat glands, collagen, and elastin (which is essential for tissue stretch and recoil). Below the dermis, the subcutaneous layer consists of loose connective tissue and fat.

Hormones exert a significant effect on skin thickness as demonstrated by the skin changes that occur during the menstrual cycle. Skin is the thinnest at the onset of the menstrual cycle when estrogens are lowest and thickens as estrogen levels rise.

Aging contributes to these hormonal changes in skin health. As we age, there is a decrease in epidermal thickness and melanocyte (pigment producing cells) concentration. In the dermis, with aging, fibroblast activity, blood vessel content, collagen, and hyaluronic acid, all decline. These changes, coupled with an increase in metalloproteinases (proteins that break down collagen), contribute to skin thinness.

Lifestyle also contributes to skin aging. Smoking and ultraviolet light exposure release inflammatory proteins that can directly damage skin by altering blood vessels and breaking down collagen.

In menopause, as estradiol levels decline, skin thickness decreases by over 1% each year for the first five years, while collagen decreases yearly by 2%. Wrinkles are caused by a reduction in elasticity secondary to loss of connective tissue which decreases 1.5% each year. Why is the face preferentially involved? Estrogen receptors are higher in the face than in the breast or thigh.

Are these skin changes reversible with estrogen supplementation? In one study, Premarin® cream, applied to the face for 24 months, produced significant increases in skin thickness and decreases in wrinkles. In a different study, 0.01% estradiol versus 0.3% estriol for six months produced no changes in systemic hormone status, but both increased skin elasticity, skin moisture, firmness, and reduced wrinkles.

If estrogen is beneficial, can its actions be enhanced by other products? Of patients given either 0.01% estradiol, or 15% glycolic acid alone or in combination, epidermal thickness was increased 23% by estradiol alone, 27% by glycolic acid alone, and 38% by both. Glycolic acid, a weak acid with small molecules that penetrate the skin easily, dissolves sebum and other substances that glue the superficial skin cells together, thus facilitating renewal of the skin surface.

Menopause is a challenge for many women. Maintaining skin's healthy appearance does not need to be part of that challenge.

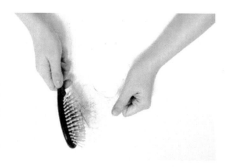

HAIR TODAY, GONE TOMORROW:
WHAT'S TESTOSTERONE GOT TO DO WITH IT?

For women in menopause, hair loss threatens one's self-image and social confidence. Termed androgenic alopecia (AGA), or "female pattern hair loss," it is misinterpreted as "going bald." Even if a woman is reassured that this is not the case, or that it affects men as well, the phenomenon evokes fear and even depression.

Under the influence of our androgens, formation of a hair begins in a follicle consisting of epidermal cells that grow down into the dermis. At the base of the follicle is the papilla, a living organ surrounded by capillaries where the hair is created and which responds to circulating hormones. As the hair forms, it grows toward the surface in a shaft of two layers, the inner layer ending below a sebaceous gland and an outer layer that attaches to the gland. The sebrum, produced by the gland, offers conditioning to the hair, which is composed of dead proteinacious material. The growth phase of normal hair (anagen phase) lasts up to three years, followed by the catagen phase (a brief intermediate period), and then a short (100 days) resting (telogen) period before the hair is discarded.

The androgen, testosterone, when converted to its active form, 5-alpha dihydrotestosterone by the enzyme 5-alpha reductase, is essential for hair on our face and body, and less for our axilla and pubic area. But age, gender, and genetics also influence this process.

In early puberty, androgens initially elicit the development of tiny vellus hairs that later become pigmented, followed by larger hairs that appear differently in different parts of the body.

The formation of 5-alpha dihydrotestosterone is key to normal hair growth. Yet excessive activity by the enzyme 5-alpha reductase produces the thinning or miniaturization of hair characteristic of AGA. In this process, over several hair cycles, there is a shortened growth or anagen phase, (a reduction from three years to 1.5 to 3 months) leading to thin, colorless hairs instead of long, firm-colored hairs. No change in number of follicles, however, occurs. If the normal growth cycle of anagen to telogen ratio is 9:1, miniaturization reduces this ratio to 2:1.

That the process is selective to certain areas of the scalp reflects the differences in embryologic origin of these scalp areas. In men and women, there is more 5-alpha reductase in frontal follicles than in occipital follicles. Additionally, women have more of the enzyme, aromatase, in the frontal and occipital scalp, which metabolizes testosterone to estrogen. Most women with AGA have normal menses. Measuring blood levels of hormones, therefore, offers little value in the evaluation. Moreover, there is no relationship of AGA to other testosterone effects on muscle, bone, or sebrum secretion.

Treatment of AGA addresses the unique aspects of this biologic event. Biotin, a water soluble B7 vitamin, improves keratin, a structural protein in hair and nails. Oral finasteride, a 5-alpha reductase type 2 inhibitor, may slow the AGA process in premenopausal but not menopausal women. Spironolactone, an aldosterone antagonist, offers mild anti-androgenic effects. Minoxidil, initially used as an antihypertensive agent, stimulates the vellus follicles. Finally, non-androgenic hair follicles transplanted from the occipital scalp to the androgen-dependent frontal areas provide a permanent solution.

Hair loss is a major insult to our sense of self-worth. Understanding the biology provides opportunities for new and innovative therapies.

MOODS AND MEMORY

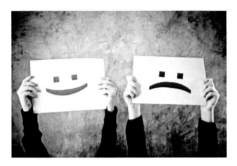

MOODS AND MENOPAUSE

There is definitely a hormonal component to our moods. This should not surprise any woman who is entering or is in menopause. The menopause transition is characterized by an initial fluctuation of estradiol production by the ovaries, evidenced by irregular menstrual cycles, but followed by a sustained estradiol decline resulting in the end of menses.

Why is estrogen important? Estrogen acts on blood vessels and neurons in many areas of the brain, but especially in the pre-frontal cortex, the center that mediates the highest level of cognitive function in primates, including humans. By stimulating the production of nitric oxide, a vasodilator, estradiol maintains blood flow to the brain. Estrogen inhibits the enzymes, monoamine oxidase and catechol-o-methyl transferase, that normally degrade and, therefore, reduce levels of serotonin, dopamine, and norepinephrine, our most important mood-altering proteins. By this enzyme-blocking action, estradiol helps to maintain a higher level of these hormones to boost and maintain our mood. Estrogen also protects our neurons from damage by oxidative free radicals and ischemic injury while helping to repair damaged nerves and stimulating growth factors to promote growth of dendritic spines (neuronal branches important for brain flexibility). This allows improved communications between neurons, which facilitates our ability to perform complex learning tasks.

What happens as the brain experiences estrogen withdrawal? From animal studies, the cognitive performance of young animals is not affected, presumably reflecting flexibility (plasticity) of the youthful brain. Older animals, in contrast, demonstrate loss in performance and, on autopsy, experience a dramatic decrease of dendritic spines. These findings correlate with human imaging studies that demonstrate decreased blood flow to the brain and actual brain shrinkage. Many women report new onset or worsening anxiety and depression at perimenopause that likely can be related to both these brain neuronal changes and life stresses. Short-term memory also can be affected by both.

Many women consider estrogen supplementation in perimenopause, not just for hot flashes and sleep disorders but also to feel better. Most current animal and human studies now are focusing on the role of estrogen replacement beginning in the perimenopausal period. Why? Initiated at this time of dramatic hormonal change in which estradiol is rapidly withdrawing and key inflammatory proteins are increasing, the benefits of estradiol protection for bone, brain, skin, and heart are more likely than if initiated late in menopause when inflammation-induced damage already has occurred.

The Women's Health Initiative Memory Study (WHIMS), one arm of the WHI, confirmed that hormone supplementation started some years after menopause did not protect against early dementia or cognitive decline. However, many believe that this study chose the wrong hormone preparations (Premarin®, made of over 12 estrogens but very little estradiol and medroxyprogesterone, a synthetic chemical version of progesterone) and the wrong age group of older women. Had they used pure estradiol with micronized progesterone, and had they studied perimenopausal women, the results would likely have been different.

Bottom Line: Many perimenopausal women report a greater sense of well-being and mood on hormone replacement therapy.

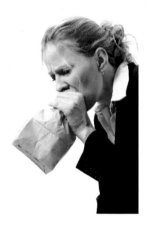

PANIC ATTACK OR GENERALIZED ANXIETY DISORDER?

Your day has been unremarkable when suddenly you experience an overwhelming sense of dread. Your heart rate begins to increase, you break into a sweat, you cannot catch your breath, your chest tightens, and you feel dizzy. You wonder, "Is this a heart attack? Is this simply anxiety? Or, have I just experienced a panic attack?"

Differentiating a panic attack from a generalized anxiety disorder can be a challenge. Generalized anxiety disorders involve chronic worry regarding a wide range of life's activities. The lifetime incidence is estimated to be 5%, with women being twice as likely as men to experience it. And while everyone at some time in his or her life has the discomfort of overwhelming anxiety, the *Diagnostic and Statistical Manual of Mental Disorders* ED V (DSM-VTR) defines generalized anxiety disorders as occurring most days within a six month window, often beginning in the teenage years and, at times, linked to alcohol or drug abuse. Typical sensations are those of restlessness, fatigue, depression, poor concentration, irritability, and negative feelings that can lead to cutting or other bodily injury as the individual seeks distraction from his or her sense of helplessness or lack of self-worth.

A panic attack, in contrast, presents as a more acute event, at times awakening a person from sleep. Officially diagnosed if experienced more than four times per month, they occur more often in women than men and may have a family predisposition. At times, the individual may even develop agoraphobia or fear of open spaces as he or she anticipates being helpless if another attack occurs.

Because of the chest tightness, high heart rate, and breathing difficulties, these episodes often are misdiagnosed initially as a cardiovascular event. The biology of panic attacks suggests a sudden fight or flight reaction to a seemingly unrecognized or ill-defined threat. The sudden release of epinephrine and norepinephrine leads to the rapid heart rate and sweating, and with the hyperventilation comes numbness and lightheadedness.

Despite the physical characteristics of panic attacks, results of numerous clinical and laboratory studies to define the specific brain regions responsible for these bodily changes have been inconclusive. They have, however, clearly defined panic attacks as a biologic process subject to pharmacologic and psychiatric management. Brain imaging and related research have demonstrated changes in oxygen, glucose, and blood flow in the limbic system and the locus ceruleus, areas that are responsible for arousal, anxiety, and fear.

Management of panic attacks in the past has utilized benzodiazepines, a family of drugs that calm the nervous system by increasing calcium channels within neurons and selective serotonin receptor inhibitors, which are antidepressants. Breathing into a bag has not been shown to be effective, whereas controlled breathing (using the 5-2-5- rhythm of five seconds to inhale, two seconds to hold one's breath, and then five seconds of slow exhale) has been shown to help. More recently, cognitive behavioral therapy has proved as effective as medications. This seemingly simple approach, where one is brought to realize that he or she cannot affect the outside world but only his or her inner response to those outside events, has proved effective as long-term therapy.

For those who have experienced panic attacks, those moments are terrifying. Our better understanding and newer approaches to treating panic attacks are providing tools for an improved life.

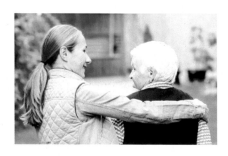

IS THERE A WINDOW FOR MENOPAUSAL HORMONE REPLACEMENT THERAPY TO HELP REDUCE THE RISK OF DEMENTIA?

Dementia conjures up many images. As we age, we all worry that the momentary misplaced car keys or the questionable location of the parked car in a large lot may indicate early dementia. In reality, the early signs of dementia are more likely evidenced by putting the car keys in the refrigerator or forgetting how to drive to your familiar home. Clinical dementia represents a group of symptoms (for example, a sore throat is a symptom) that can have many causes, including infection, e.g., human immunodeficiency virus (HIV), vascular diseases, stroke, Huntington's disease, Parkinson's disease, and Alzheimer's disease. Dementia is formally characterized by a progressive decline in multiple brain functions including memory, cognitive function, and reasoning.

The incidence of dementia is staggering. Progressive Alzheimer's disease consists of loss of memory, along with declines in language, spatial orientation, and personality, and is the cause of 60% of dementia. While dementia is rare for those under 65 years, its incidence doubles every five years and affects over one-third of individuals over 85 years. Estimates from the National Institutes of Health (NIH) are that more than five million Americans suffer from this disease.

The biology of Alzheimer's disease is now better understood, but prevention remains an unsolved target. Alzheimer's disease symptoms likely result from deposition of the protein, hypophosphorylated tau, within the microtubules inside nerve cells of the brain, causing fibril tangles, and also the laying down of B-amyloid, a neurotoxin, between these cells. This process interferes with communication between brain cells, leading to cell death with eventual brain shrinkage. Early onset Alzheimer's disease (diagnosed under 60 years) makes up only 5% of the affected population and is transmitted like an autosomal dominant trait, while the vast majority of late onset patients have some combination of genetic, environmental, and lifestyle factors. The presentation of early versus late Alzheimer's disease appears to depend partly upon mutations in the encoding apolipoprotein e gene (APOE), a lipid transport protein important for normal neural function and repair of damaged neurons.

Because dementia is diagnosed more frequently in women than in men and begins in midlife, logic would suggest a link between dementia and declining gonadal hormones, especially estradiol. Clinical and animal studies and in-vitro analyses support this premise. The concept that estradiol could influence cognition is evidenced as ovarian production of estradiol begins to decline two to three years before onset of menopause (a period called the menopause transition) when women may notice a decline in episodic memory, often accompanied by anxiety or depression. This phenomenon appears to accelerate in postmenopausal women who are not on hormone replacement. In-vitro and animal studies indicate that estradiol enhances activity at neuronal synapses, neuronal growth, and the ability of the hippocampus to grow new cells needed for episodic memory. Moreover, estradiol has been shown to protect against neural injury from ischemia, reactive oxygen species, and other excitatory toxins.

These combined data provide strong support that menopausal estradiol replacement might reduce the risk of Alzheimer's disease. To address this question, the Women's Health Initiative Memory Study (WHIMS) was initiated in 1996. The study selected only women over 65 years to assure an adequate number that would develop dementia over the course of the study. After six years of follow-up, however, those on conjugated equine estradiol (CEE) and medroxyprogesterone or CEE alone fared worse than those on a placebo. Subsequent analysis has challenged these conclusions based on medication choice and how the patients were distributed in the study. Nonetheless, the investigators concluded that estrogen given to older women does not reduce, and perhaps may increase, the risk of dementia.

Current recommendations are that hormone supplementation for menopausal symptoms should be started in the late 40s or early 50s (early menopause) in order to decrease the risk of osteoporosis and cardiovascular disease. Extension of this opinion would suggest that there may be a window of opportunity for hormone supplementation to reduce Alzheimer's risk. Estradiol has been shown in-vitro to decrease B-amyloid formation, reduce hypophosphorylation of tau proteins, and increase apolipoprotein expression. Moreover, several smaller studies have demonstrated a decline in dementia risk in those who began hormone replacement early in menopause and also those who have taken hormone supplementation sometime in the past. Indeed, it may be that estradiol can help protect healthy brain cells but can accelerate adverse changes in already diseased ones.

The impact of hormone supplementation to reduce the risk of dementia remains controversial. Nonetheless, initiating hormone replacement in early menopause is rapidly gaining support as newer studies concentrate on treating younger women to preserve their cognition later in life.

BREAST CANCER

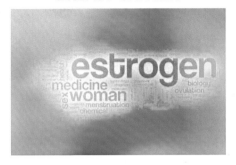

ESTROGEN AND BREAST CANCER: A LOVE-HATE RELATIONSHIP

What do the dates 1896 and 1935 have to do with breast cancer? They mark critical moments in clarifying the complex relationship between estrogen and breast cancer. Breast cancer is the second leading cause of cancer mortality in the United States and Canada. Understanding its relationship to estrogen is critical for attributing cause and planning future therapies.

In 1896, it was observed that breast cancer regressed if women had .both ovaries removed (surgical menopause) or progressed into natural menopause, even though estrogen had not yet been discovered as a hormone. In 1916, this relationship was demonstrated in the animal model, and in 1923 estrogen was identified and named.

Clinical studies reinforced the concept that length of estrogen exposure affected breast cancer risk. Risk factors include women with early onset menses or late menopause, women who do not have children or who have had children later in life, women who do not breastfeed, obese women, and those who abuse alcohol. The estrogen-induced biologic pathway leading to breast cancer has been shown to involve estrogen-related gene mutations and generation of reactive oxygen species.

At odds with this process is the fact that in The Women's Health

Initiative (WHI) report of 2002, women with a hysterectomy who were given only conjugated estrogen (Premarin®) and not the combination of Premarin® and the synthetic progestin, medroxyprogesterone acetate (as PremPro®), showed a reduction in breast cancer incidence and mortality compared to controls. It appears that under certain circumstances, estrogen protects against breast cancer. How could this be?

Haddo, a British microbiologist, first demonstrated in his laboratory that under certain circumstances some synthetic estrogens, one being diethylstilbestrol (DES), can retard growth of breast cancer cells and later confirmed this finding in a clinical trial. By the 1960s, DES in high doses was being used to treat breast cancer, producing a reduction in breast cancer cells in one-third of women. However, for breast cancer survivors at least five years into menopause and therefore deprived of estrogen for an extended period, estrogen's action to kill breast cancer cells was more striking than that for younger women.

The science of breast cancer is changing continuously. Evidence is accruing that while breast cancer in most cases does involve a lifetime of estrogen exposure, if those breast cancer cells are deprived of estrogen for an extended period, they change, and estrogen then becomes a "lethal bullet." This concept appears radical but in time may provide new approaches to the treatment of breast cancer.

⬚⬚

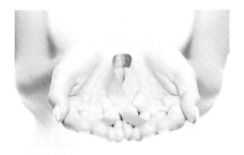

IS ALL BREAST CANCER THE SAME?

Most women are aware of a link between estrogen and breast cancer. Yet, there are different types of breast cancer i.e., ductal, lobular, inflammatory, with various receptor characteristics that guide treatment. Approximately 75% of breast cancer is estrogen receptor (ER) positive. However, there are conditions in which estrogen both fuels and at other times kills ER-positive breast cancer cells. One type of breast cancer does not even recognize estrogen at all. In 2011, there were 230,480 new cases of breast cancer and 57,650 cases of breast carcinoma in situ while 29,520 women were predicted to die of this disease. Understanding the types of breast cancer offers promise for improved surveillance, prevention and more effective treatments.

Observers noted as early as 1896 that the ovaries were related to breast cancer since some women with breast cancer improved after their ovaries were removed. Yet, it was not until 1923 that estrogen as a hormone was discovered. While estrogen can stimulate growth of certain breast cancer cells, if these cells are deprived of hormones for five years by anti-estrogen medication, they are made vulnerable to being killed by estrogen through cell apoptosis. This may explain the cancer-killing effect of diethylstilbesterol (DES) in the 1960s when one third of women with breast cancer given the drug improved.

Duration of exposure to estrogen over a woman's lifetime relates to the risk for developing estrogen-receptor positive breast cancer. This form of breast cancer is more common in women with early onset menses, late onset menopause, and nulliparity or having children later in life. All of these situations involve prolonged menstrual cycling and estrogen exposure. Other risk factors are lack of breastfeeding, alcohol consumption (which increases estrogen production) and obesity, since adipose cells produce estrogen. Additional factors are smoking, family history, and genetic status.

The association of ER-positive breast cancer to lifelong estrogen exposure helps explain why such women are usually older at cancer onset. In the Women's Health Initiative (WHI), the average age of participants was 63. Estrogen in the form of Premarin plus the synthetic progestin, medroxyprogesterone (PremPro), given to women who still had their uterus, increased overall breast cancer risk. Yet, in women without a uterus, estrogen replacement therapy alone (ERT) decreased the overall breast cancer risk. Whether the synthetic progestin in the first group contributed to the increase in breast cancer remains unclear. In the second group, estrogen was not started until nearly 10 years after menopause, so a period of estrogen deprivation preceding the estrogen-only exposure may have induced apoptosis of nascent cancer cells.

Certain other breast cancers do not express the common hormone receptor genes for estrogen, progesterone or the newer marker, human epidermal growth factor (HER2). Called triple-negative breast cancer (TNBC), this cancer, first reported in 2005, often occurs in younger women, even during their reproductive years, and appears to be more aggressive. In one study, 33.8% of women under 40 with breast cancer were TNBC, while only 21.5% were ER positive. Yet, for all types of breast cancer, 23.9% of women were younger, while 76.1% were older.

Understanding the characteristics of these breast cancers challenges current protocols for surveillance and management. Controversy exists as to when to begin providing mammography to women. Administering estrogen after five years of anti-estrogen treatment may provide additional protection for ER-positive breast cancer survivors. In fact, ongoing studies of anti-estrogen treatment alternating with ERT or "drug holidays" may answer some of these questions. Medical science is built on questions leading to answers that ask more questions. Progress in breast cancer research exemplifies this process.

◻◻

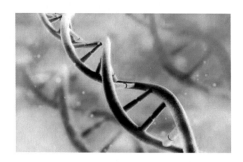

BRCA GENES: PROTECTOR FROM OR CAUSE OF BREAST CANCER?

Many women have heard of the term "BRCA" standing for Breast Cancer Associated genes and their association with inherited breast cancers. Perhaps not as well-known is the fact that the BRCA genes normally play an important role in protecting our bodies as they age. It is only when mutations of these BRCA genes occur that the risk for developing cancer increases, because the mutations inactivate their protective effects.

Throughout our lifetime, our body continually is engaged in renewing itself. Every minute, somewhere in our body our aging cells pass on their "personality" by creating "daughter cells" that will replace them in location and function. Old cardiac cells produce identical but younger heart cells. Old muscle cells generate newer muscle cells and so on. These amazing events occur through a process called deoxyribonucleic acid (DNA) replication.

The genetic makeup for each cell in our body is contained in a double-stranded DNA molecule. Each time a cell divides, the two resulting daughter cells each receive the same genetic information that was contained in the DNA of the parent cell, but it is the organization of the DNA that gives it its genomic identity. The two strands of the DNA, which provide the backbone of the molecule, are connected by bonding of strand components called nucleotides, arranged like steps on a ladder. The nucleotides, adenine (A) and thymine (T), always pair with one another, as do the nucleotides, cytosine (C) and guanine (G). The specific arrangement of these pairs of nucleotides along the double-stranded DNA, like a computer code, produces the unique genetic fingerprint of that cell.

The process by which daughter cells are provided the identical genetic makeup of the parent cell begins as the two DNA strands in the parent cell are separated, much as a zipper is unzipped, leaving each strand with its own complement of half paired nucleotides, bearing all necessary information to make a new cell. While each strand is open, free-floating nucleotides present in the cellular environment that normally pair with those specific nucleotides are secured, thus reestablishing the paired relationship. Finally, enzymes reassemble the new strands into a double-coiled arrangement in each of the daughter cells. Since each time a cell divides it has to copy and transmit the exact sequence of more than three billion nucleotides to its daughter cells, it is easy to understand the risks of transmitting mistakes to the next generation of cells.

It is in the governing of this process that BRCA genes normally play an important role. DNA replication occurs in an orderly fashion dictated by progression through a cell cycle made up of five steps designated G0 (resting), G1 (first gap), S (synthesis), G2 (second gap), and M (mitosis) phases. Each phase is separated by a checkpoint in which transition from one step to the next mandates that all requirements at that checkpoint are satisfied. If at any checkpoint problems are encountered, the cell cycle is stopped until repairs are made. The undamaged BRCA genes oversee this repair process.

There are five known repair pathways which can be activated when ultraviolet light, cosmic or isotopic irradiation, environmental pollution, cigarette smoking, or other insults damage our DNA. Two important mechanisms are homologous recombination repair (HRR) and non-homologous enjoining (NHEJ). BRCA genes participate in both, specializing in the rejoining of double-stranded DNA that has been cut clean through, leaving the chromosome in two pieces. Non-homologous enjoining ligates DNA damaged ends in G1 phase by removing or adding bases to the broken ends. Homologous recombination repair only functions at the checkpoint between S and G2. Rejoining broken chromosomal DNA suppresses the uncontrolled replication of breast cells leading to a malignant tumor.

Inherited mutations of the BRCA1 and BRCA2 genes, identified in 1990 and 1995 respectively, inactivate the repair capacity of the genes, removing this protective shield. Significantly, since inherited BRCA mutations come from the germ line that is the source of all cells in the body, they greatly increase cancer risk. In the case of breast cells, all have the mutation, and so all are impaired in DNA strand joining.

The clinical implications have been recognized only recently. Today, in the general population, there is a 12% lifetime risk for breast cancer, yet by age 70 there is a 55% to 65% risk of breast cancer if one carries a BRCA1 mutation and a 45% risk with a BRCA2 mutation. Lifetime risk for ovarian cancer in the general population is 1.3%, but 39% of women with the BRCA1 mutations and 11% to 17% with the BRCA2 mutations will develop ovarian cancer by age 70.

How has this information helped women? Advances in cancer management have resulted from risk identity, improved surveillance, and targeted treatments. Genetic research and engineering, as well as expanding our knowledge of the health and risks to our DNA, focus on all three areas of science.

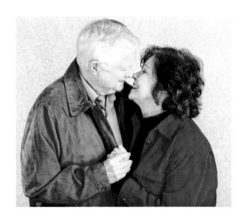

INTIMACY AND THE BREAST CANCER SURVIVOR

Early detection and directed treatments have led to improved outcomes for women with breast cancer. Nonetheless, the gynecologic impact of these treatments is significant. In one study, 42% of breast cancer survivors experienced vaginal dryness, 38% reported that intercourse was painful, and 64% felt loss of libido. For many women, these changes affect her relationship with her partner directly, thereby increasing her risk of depression. Furthermore, medical treatment for depression can accelerate loss of sexual interest and further endanger the relationship. In one series, when 610 breast cancer survivors with normal sexual activity were given antidepressants, 57% experienced loss of libido.

For menopausal women without breast cancer, systemic or vaginal estrogens have been the treatment of choice for vaginal dryness and pain during intercourse. The dilemma facing the breast cancer survivor is that in vitro, animal, and human clinical studies document that long-term estrogen exposure is linked to the development, progression, and recurrence of breast cancer. In fact, aromatase inhibitors and tamoxifen, which block estrogen, often are used prophylactically for five to ten years after immediate breast cancer treatment. Consistent with this anti-estrogen approach, the medical community has been forced to adopt a "no hormone for you" stance for breast cancer survivors.

Efforts to evaluate the role of vaginal estrogen for breast cancer survivors have produced mixed results, but at least one small study has reported that vaginal estrogen in certain women can elevate circulating blood estrogen levels above that observed normally in menopause. Are there other approaches? Vaginal testosterone and DHEA creams have been tested clinically, and neither increases the circulating levels of estrogen above menopausal levels. The biologic benefits draw from the fact that the androgens applied to the vagina are not acting through an androgen receptor but most likely are being converted to estrogens at the local tissue level. Nonetheless, monitoring estrogen blood levels is a critical part of this management. Neither, however, is FDA approved for this purpose currently.

Most patients using either of these androgen creams experience less vaginal dryness, a lower vaginal pH, and increased moisture. Water-based gels are available if the vehicle used in the compounded androgen cream or gel generates local irritation. Many of these women again find intercourse less uncomfortable.

Survivors of breast cancer treatment have a very challenging journey made more complicated by the fact that many of these treatments have an impact on the couple's relationship. This new information about the use of androgens for treating vaginal dryness and pain on intercourse for breast cancer survivors does not address all of the symptoms of treatment-induced menopause, but it provides some local solutions to vaginal dryness and pain.

REFERENCES AND RELATED READINGS

GENERAL DISCUSSION

INTRODUCTION

American College of Obstetricians and Gynecologists (2014). ACOG practice bulletin no. 141: Management of Menopausal Symptoms. Obstetrics and Gynecology, 123(1):202-216.

Harlow SD, Gass M, Hall JE, Lobo R, Maki P, Rebar RW, Sherman S, Sluss PM, and de Villiers TJ (2012). Executive summary of the stages of Reproductive Aging Workshop + 10: Addressing the unfinished agenda of staging reproductive aging. Menopause, 19:1-9.

NAMS Practice Pearl; Extended duration use of menopausal hormone therapy (2013). 1-5.

Position Statement; the 2012 Hormone therapy position statement of the North American Menopause Society (2012). Menopause, 19:57-271.

Rossouw JE, Manson JE, Kaunitz AM, and Anderson GL (2013). Lessons learned from the women's health initiative trials of menopausal hormone therapy. Obstetrics and Gynecology, 121;172-176.

Shifren JL and Gass MLS (2014). The North American Menopause Society Recommendations for Clinical Care of Midlife Women. Menopause, 21:125.

THE PUBLIC FACE OF MENOPAUSE

No references. Personal observations.

UNDERSTANDING MENOPAUSE (AT THE MOST BASIC LEVEL)

Harlow SD, Gass M, Hall JE, Lobo R, Maki P, Rebar RW, Sherman S, Sluss PM, and de Villiers TJ (2012). Executive summary of the stages of Reproductive Aging Workshop + 10: Addressing the unfinished agenda of staging reproductive aging. Menopause, 19:1-9.

Matthews KA, Crawford SL, Chae CU, Everson-Rose SA, Sowers MF, Sternfeld B, and Sutton-Tyrrell K (2009). Are changes in cardiovascular disease risk factors in midlife women due to chronological aging or to the menopausal transition? Journal of the American College of Cardiology, 54:2366-2373.

Pfeilschifter J, Koditz R, Pfohl M, and Schatz H (2002). Changes in proinflammatory cytokine activity after menopause. Endocrine Reviews, 23:90-199.

Straub RH (2007). The complex role of estrogens in inflammation. Endocrine Reviews, 28:521-574.

Takao T, Kumagai C, Hisakawa N, Matsumoto R, ands Hashimoto K (2005). Effect of 17-B-estradiol on tumor necrosis factor-alpha-induced cytotoxicity in the human peripheral T lymphocyte. Journal of Endocrinology, 184:191-197.

WHY IS MENOPAUSE MANAGEMENT NOT BETTER UNDERSTOOD BY OB/GYN PROVIDERS?

No references. Personal observations.

CLARIFYING THE TERMS "BIOIDENTICAL HORMONES" AND "COMPOUNDED HORMONES"

Fugh-Berman A and Bythrow J (2007). Bioidentical hormones for menopausal hormone therapy: Variation on a theme. Journal of General Internal Medicine, 22:1030-1034.

McCormick K (2012). Compounded bioidentical hormones. Connections: An Educational Resource of Women's International Pharmacy, (2012) 1-6.

Moskowitz D (2006). A comprehensive review of the safety and efficacy of bioidentical hormones for the management of menopause and related health risks. Alternative Medicine Review, 11:208-223.

WAS THE WOMEN'S HEALTH INITIATIVE GOOD OR BAD FOR WOMEN'S HEALTH?

Ochnik, AM, Moore NL, Jankovic-Karasoulos T, Bianco-Miotto T, Ryan NK, Thomas MR, Birrell SN, Burler LM, Tilley WD, and Hickey TE (2013). Antiandrogenic actions of medroxyprogesterone acetate on epithelial cells within normal human breast tissues cultured ex vivo. Menopause, 21:79-88.

Rossouw JE, Manson JE, Kaunitz AM, and Anderson GL (2013). Lessons learned from the women's health initiative trials of menopausal hormone therapy. Obstetrics and Gynecology, 121:172-176.

Simon JA (2014). What if the Women's Health Initiative had used transdermal estradiol and oral progesterone instead? Menopause, a21:769-783.

SPICE, PICKLES FOR LEG CRAMPS. CAN IT BE THAT SIMPLE?

Abdulla AJ, Jones PW, Pearce VR. Leg cramps in the elderly: prevalence, drug and disease association. Int J Clin Pract. (1999) 53;494-496.

Butler JV, Mulkerrin EC, O'Keeffe ST. Nocturnal leg cramps in older people. Postgradmed. (2002) 78: 596-598.

Futterman M. A new way to prevent muscle cramps. The wall Street Journal July 11, 2016.

Miller KC, Mack GW, KNigh KL, Hopkins JT, Draper DO, Fields PJ, Henter I. Reflex inhibition of electrically induced muscle cramps in hypohydrated humans. Med Sci Sports Exerc (2010) 42; 953-61.

Miller KCC. Elecrolyte and plasma responses after pickle juice, mustard, and deionized water ingestion in dehydrated humans. J Athle Train (2014) 49; 360-7.

Naylor RJ, Young JB. A general population survey of leg cramps. Age Ageing (1994) 23;418-20.

I'M GETTING OLDER... AM I STILL RELEVANT?

No references. Personal observations.

HORMONE BIOLOGY

THE STORY OF ESTROGEN: NOT JUST YOUR MOTHER'S HORMONE

Canonico M (2014). Hormone therapy and hemostasis among postmenopausal women: A review. Menopause, 21:753-762.

Canonico M, Plu-Bureau, Lowe GD, and Scarabin P-Y (2008). Hormone replacement and risk of venous thromboembolism in postmenopausal women: Systematic review and meta-analysis. BMJ, 31:1227-1231.

Cushman M (2010). Patch instead of pill: A safer menopausal estrogen? Journal of the American Heart Association: Arteriosclerosis, Thrombosis, and Vascular Biology. 30:136-137.

Gross CG (1998). Claude Bernard and the consistency of the internal environment. The Neuroscientist, 4:380-385.

Shufelt, CL, Merz, CNB, Prentice, RL, Pettinger, MB, Rossouw, JE, Aroda, VR, Kaunitz, AM, Lakshminarayan, K, Martin, LW, Phillips, LS and Manson, JE (2014). Hormone therapy dose, formulation, route of delivery, and risk of cardiovascular events in women: Findings from the Women's Health Initiative Observational Study. Menopause, 21:260-266.Tara JR (2005).

One hundred years of hormones, EMBO Reports, 6:490-496.

Vance DA (20047). Premarin: The intriguing history of a controversial drug. International Journal of Pharaceutical Compounding, 11:282-286.

Watson MC (1935). Observations on the treatment of dysmenorrhea with the placental extract "Emmenin." The Canadian Medical Association Journal, 32:609-614.

FROM MENARCHE TO MENOPAUSE: THE STORY OF PROGESTERONE

Corner GW. The early history of progesterone. Gynecol Invest (1974) 5; 106-112.

Levy T, Yairi Y, Bar-Hava I, Shalev J, Orvieto R, Ben-Rafael Z. Pharmacokinetics of the progesterone-containing vaginal tablet and its use in assisted reproduction. Steroids (2000) 65; 645-649.

R A Wilson. Birth Control, Pills and Menopause Prevention. In Feminine Forever (1966) Chapter 9; 178-193. Pocket Books NY.

Simon JA. What if the Women's Health Initiative had used transdermal estradiol and oral progesterone instead? Menopause (2014) 7; 769-783.

Stefanick ML. Estrogens and progestins: background and history, trends in use, and guidelines and regimes approved by the US Food and Drug Administration. Am J of Med (2005) 118; 64S-73S.

Tata JR. One hundred years of hormones. EMBO reports (2005) 6; 490-496.

Tavaniotou A, Smitz J, Bourgain C, Devroey Pl Comparison between different routes of progesterone administration as luteal phase support in infertility treatments. Hum Reprod Update (2000) 6; 139-48.

The "Marker Degradation" and creation of the Mexican steroid hormone industry 1938-1945. University Park, Pennsylvania (1999) American Chemical Society.

Writing Group for the Women's Health Initiative Investigators. Risks and benefits of estrogen plus progestin in healthy postmenopausal women. JAMA express (2002) 288; 321-333.

THE PILL OR THE PATCH: ARE ALL ESTROGENS THE SAME?

Cananova G and Spritzer PM (2012). Effects of micronized progesterone added to non-oral estradiol on lipids and cardiovascular risk factors in early postmenopause: A clinical trial. Lipids in Health and Disease, 11:133-140.

Canonico M, Oger E, Plu-Bureau G, Conard J, Meyer G, Levesque H, Trillot N, Barrellier M-T, Wahl D, Emmerich J, and Scarabin P-Y (2007). Hormone therapy and venous thromboembolism among postmenopausal women: Impact of the route of estrogen administration and progestogens: the ESTHER study. Circulation, 115:840-845.

Custham M (2010). Patch instead of pill: A safer menopausal estrogen? Artherosclerosis, thrombosis, and vascular biology. Journal of the American Heart Association, 30:136-137.

Liu B (2013). Is transdermal menopausal hormone therapy a safer option than oral therapy? Canadian Medical Association Journal, 185:549-550.

Miler VM, Black DM, Brinton EA, Budoff MJ, Cedars MI, Hodis HN, Lobo RA, Manson JE, Merriam GR, Naftolin F, Santoro N, Taylor HS, and Harman SM (2009). Using basic science to design a clinical trial: Baseline characteristics of women enrolled in the Kronos Early Estrogen Prevention study (KEEPS). Journal of Cardiovascular Translational Research, 2:228-239.

Raz L, Hunter LW, Jayachandran M, Heit JA, and Miller VM (2014). Differential effects of oral and transdermal menopausal hormone therapy on prostacyclin and thromboxane in platelets. Physiological Reports, 2:e00275-e00285.

Renoux C, Dell'Aniello S, Garbe E, Suissa S (2009). Transdermal and oral hormone replacement therapy and the risk of stroke. A nested casecontrol study. BMJ, 3:340-347.

PROGRESS IN SAFETY OF HORMONE DELIVERY

Canonico M, Plu-Bureau, Lowe GD, and Scarabin P-Y (2008). Hormone replacement and risk of venous thromboembolism in postmenopausal women: Systematic review and meta-analysis. BMJ, 31:1227-1231.

Canonico M (2014). Hormone therapy and hemostasis among postmenopausal women: A review. Menopause, 21:753-762.

Cushman M (2010). Patch instead of pill: A safer menopausal estrogen? Journal of the American Heart Association: Arteriosclerosis, Thrombosis, and Vascular Biology. 30:136-137.

Shufelt, CL, Merz, CNB, Prentice, RL, Pettinger, MB, Rossouw, JE, Aroda, VR, Kaunitz, AM, Lakshminarayan, K, Martin, LW, Phillips, LS and Manson, JE (2014). Hormone therapy dose, formulation, route of delivery, and risk of cardiovascular events in women: Findings from the Women's Health Initiative Observational Study. Menopause, 21:260-266.

UPDATE ON TIMING OF HORMONE REPLACEMENT THERAPY IN MENOPAUSE

American College of Obstetricians and Gynecologists (2014). ACOG practice bulletin no. 141: Management of Menopausal Symptoms. Obstetrics and Gynecology, 123(1):202-216.

Avis NE, Crawford SL, Greendale G, Bromberger JT, Everson-Rose SA, Gold EB, Hess R, Joffe H, Kravitz HM, Tepper PG, and Thruston RC (2015). Duration of menopausal vasomotor symptoms over the menopause transition. Journal of the American Medical Association, 175(4):531-539.

Crandall CJ, Tseng C-H, Crawford SL, Thurston RC, Gold EB, Johnston JM, and Greendale GA (2011). Association of menopausal vasomotor symptoms with increased bone turnover during the menopausal transition. Journal of Bone and Mineral Research, 26:840-849.

Kaunitz AM and Manson JAE (2015). Failure to treat menopausal symptoms: A disconnect between clinical practice and scientific data. Menopause, 22:687-688.

Kaunitz AM (2014). Extended duration of use of menopausal hormone therapy. Menopause, 21(6):679-681.

Pinkerton JAV (2015). Money talks: Untreated hot flashes cost women, the workplace and society. Editorial. Menopause, 22:254-255.

Politi MC, Schleinitz MD, and Col NF (2008). Revising the duration of vasomotor symptoms of menopause: A meta-analysis. Journal of General Internal Medicine, 23:1507-1513.

Sarrel P, Portman D, Lefebvre P, Lafeuille M-H, Grittner AM, Fortier J, Gravel J, Duh MS, and Aupperle PM (2015). Incremental direct and indirect costs of untreated vasomotor symptoms. Menopause, 22:260-266.

Thurston RC, El Khoudary SR, Sutton-Tyrrell K, Crandall CJ, Gold E, Sternfeld B, Selzer F, and Matthews KA (2011). Are vasomotor symptoms associated with alterations in hemostatic and inflammatory markers? Findings from the study of women's health across the nation. Menopause, 18:1044-1051.

MENOPAUSE OR MENOPAUSE TRANSITION:
WHEN DOES THE BIOLOGY BEGIN?

Harlow SD, Gass M, Hall JE, Lobo R, Maki P, Rebar RW, Sherman S, Sluss PM, and de Villiers TJ (2012). Executive summary of the stages of Reproductive Aging Workshop + 10: Addressing the unfinished agenda of staging reproductive aging. Menopause, 19:1-9.

Lobo RA (2008). Metabolic syndrome after menopause and the role of hormones. Maturitas, 60:10-18.

Lovejoy JC, Champagne CM, de Jonge L, Xie H, and Smith SR (2008). Increased visceral fat and decreased energy expenditure during the menopausal transition. International Journal of Obesity, 32:949-958.

Matthews KA, Crawford SL, Chae CU, Everson-Rose SA, Sowers MF, Sternfeld B, and Sutton-Tyrrell K (2009). Are changes in cardiovascular disease risk factors in midlife women due to chronological aging or to the menopausal transition? Journal of the American College of Cardiology, 54:2366-2373.

MENOPAUSE TRANSITION: DON'T MISS THIS
IMPORTANT PREVENTATIVE HEALTH OPPORTUNITY

Abel ED, O'Shea M, Ramasamy R. Insulin Resistance: metabolic mechanisms and consequences in the heart. Arteriosclerosis, Thrombosis, and Vascular Biology (2012) 32;2068-2076.

Betra A, Siegmund B. The role of visceral fat. Dig Dis (2012) 30;70-4.

Chistiakov DA, Bobryshev YV, Kozarov E, Sobenin IA, Orekhov AN. Role of gut microbiota in the modulation of atherosclerosis-associated immune response. Frontiers in Microbiology (2015) 6; 1-7.

Clark G, Stilling RM, Kennedy PJ, Stanton C, Cryan JF, Dinan TG. Mol Endocrino (2014) 28; 1221-1238.

Forbes JD, Domselaar GV, Bernstein CN. The gut microbiota immune-mediated inflammatory diseases. Frontiers in Microbiology (2016) 7;1-18.

Frayn KN. Visceral fat and insulin-resistance-causative or correlative? Br J Nutr (2000) 83; s71-77.

Hanauer S. Obesity and visceral fat: a growing inflammatory disease. Nature Clinical Practice; Gastroenterology and Hepatology (2005) 2; 245.

Klein S. The case of visceral fat: argument for the defense. JCI (2004) 11; 1530-1532.

Kredel LI, Siegmund B. Adipose-tissue and intestinal inflammation-visceral obesity and creeping fat. Frontiers of Immunology (2014) 5; 462-73.

Lobo RA. Metabolic syndrome after menopause and the role of hormones. Maturitas (2008) 60; 10-18.

Nielsen S, Guo Z, Johnson CM, Hensrud DD, Jensen MD. Splanchnic lipolysis in human obesity. JCI (2004) 113; 1582-88.

Forbes JD, Domselaar GV, Bernstein CN. The gut microbiota immune-mediated inflammatory diseases. Frontiers in Microbiology (2016) 7;1-18.

Petschow B, Dore J, Hibberd P, Dinan T, et al. Probiotics, prebiotics and the host microbiome: the science of translation. Annals of the new York Academy of Sciences (2013) 1306;1-17.

Shuster A, Patlas M, Pinthus JH, Mourtzakis M. The clinical importance of visceral adiposity: a critical review of methods for visceral adipose tissue analysis. Br J of Radiology (2012) 85; 1-10.

Yki-Jarvinen H. Liver fat in the pathogenesis of insulin resistance and type 2 diabetes. Dig Dis (2010) 28l; 203-9.

HOT FLASHES

WHAT DO WE KNOW ABOUT HOT FLASHES IN MENOPAUSE?

American College of Obstetricians and Gynecologists (2014). ACOG practice bulletin no. 141: Management of Menopausal Symptoms. Obstetrics and Gynecology, 123(1):202-216.

Avis NE, Crawford SL, Greendale G, Bromberger JT, Everson-Rose SA, Gold EB, Hess R, Joffe H, Kravitz HM, Tepper PG, and Thruston RC (2015). Duration of Menopausal Vasomotor Symptoms over the Menopause Transition. Journal of the American Medical Association, 175:531-539.

Butt DA, Lock M, Lewis JE, Ross S, and Moineddin R (2008). Gabapentin for the treatment of menopausal hot flashes: A randomized controlled trial. Menopause, 15:310-318.

Carrol DG (2006). Non hormonal therapies for hot flashes in menopause. American Family Physician, 73:457-464.

Crandall CJ, Tseng C-H, Crawford SL, Thurston RC, Gold EB, Johnston JM, and Greendale GA (2011). Association of menopausal vasomotor symptoms with increased bone turnover during the menopausal transition. Journal of Bone and Mineral Research, 26:840-849.

Freeman EW, Guthrie KA, Caan B, Sternfeld B, Cohen LS, Joffe H, Carpenter JS, Anderson GL, Larson JC, Ensrud KE, Reed SD, Newton KM, Sherman S, Sammel MD, and LaCroix AZ (2011). Efficacy of Escitalopram for hot flashes in healthy menopausal women. Journal of the American Medical Association, 305:267-274.

Freedman RR (2001). Physiology of hot flashes. American Journal of Human Biology, 13:453-464.

Grady D (2015). Management of Menopausal Symptoms. New England Journal of Medicine, 355:2338-2347.

Guthrie KA, LaCroix AZ, Ensrud KE, Joffe H, Newton KM, Reed SD, Caan B, Carpenter JS, Cohen LS, Freeman EW, Larson JC, Manson JE, Rexrode K, Skaar TC, Sternfeld B, and Anderson GL (2015). Pooled analysis of six pharmacologic and nonpharmacologic interventions for vasomotor symptoms. Obstetrics and Gynecology, 126:413-422.

Joffe H, Guthrie KA, LaCroix AZ, Reed SD, Ensrud KE, Manson JE, Newton KM, Freeman EW, Anderson GL, Larson JC, Hunt J, Shifren J, Rexrode KM, Caan B, Sternfeld B, Carpenter JS, and Cohen L (2014). Low-dose estradiol and the serotonin-norepinephrine reuptake inhibitor Venlafaxine for vasomotor symptoms: A randomized clinical trial. Journal of the American Medical Association, 174:1058-1066.

Kaunitz AM and Manson JAE (2015). Failure to treat menopausal symptoms: A disconnect between clinical practice and scientific data. Menopause, 22:687-688.

Morrow PKH, Mattair DN, and Hortobagyi GN (2011). Hot Flashes: A review of pathophysiology and treatment modalities. The Oncologist, 16:16581664.

Nelson HD (2004). Commonly used types of postmenopausal estrogen for treatment of hot flashes. Journal of the American Medical Association, 291:1610-1620.

Pandya KJ, Morrow GR, Roscoe JA, Zhao H, Hickok JT, Pajon E, Sweeney TJ, Banerjee TK, and Flynn PJ (2005). Gabapentin for hot flashes in 420 women with breast cancer: A randomized double-blind placebo-controlled trial. Lancet, 366(9488):818-824.

Pinkerton JAV (2015). Money talks: untreated hot flashes cost women, the workplace and society. Editorial. <u>Menopause</u>, 22:254-255.

Politi MC, Schleinitz MD, and Col NF (2008). Revising the duration of vasomotor symptoms of menopause: A meta-analysis. <u>Journal of General Internal Medicine</u>, 23:1507-1513.

Sarrel P, Portman D, Lefebvre P, Lafeuille M-H, Grittner AM, Fortier J, Gravel J, Duh MS, and Aupperle PM (2015). Incremental direct and indirect costs of untreated vasomotor symptoms. <u>Menopause</u>, 22:260-266.

Shams T, Firwana B, Habib F, Alshahrani A, Ainouh B, Murad MH, and Ferwana M (2007). SSRIS for hot flashes: A systematic review and metaanalysis of randomized trials. <u>Journal of General Internal Medicine</u>, 29:204213.

Sideras K and Loprinzi C (2010). Nonhormonal management of hot flashes for women on risk reduction therapy. <u>Journal of the National Comprehensive Cancer Network</u>, 8:1171-1179.

Simon JA, Portman DJ, Kaunitz AM, Mekonnen H, Kazempour K, Bhaskar S, and Lippman J (2013). Low-dose paroxetine 7.5 mg for menopausal vasomotor symptoms: two randominzed controlled trials. <u>Menopause</u>, 20:1027-1035.

Thurston RC and Joffe H (2011). Vasomotor symptoms and menopause: Findings from the Study of Women's Health Across the Nation. <u>Obstetrics and Gynecology Clinics of North America</u>, 38:489-501.

HOT FLASH CONNECTION TO PUBERTY

McCarthy MM (2013). A piece in the puzzle of puberty. <u>Nature Neuroscience</u>, 16:251-253.

De Tassigny D and Colledge WH (2010). The role of kisspeptin signaling in reproduction. <u>Physiology</u>, 25:207-217.

Freedman RR (2001). Physiology of hot flashes. <u>American Journal of Human Biology</u>, 13:453-464.

Grady D (2015). Management of Menopausal Symptoms. <u>New England Journal of Medicine</u> 355:2338-2347.

Han SK, Gottsch ML, Lee KJ, Popa SM, Smith JT, Jakawich SK, Clifton DK, Steiner RA, and Herbison AE (2005). Activation of gonadotrophin-related hormone neurons by Kisspeptin as a neuroendocrine switch for the onset of puberty. <u>The Journal of Neuroscience</u>, 25:11349-11356.

Hrabovszky E (2014). Neuroanatomy of the human hypothalamic kisspeptin system. Neuroendocrinology, 99:33-49.

Mittelman-Smith MA, Krajewski-Hall SJ, McMullen NT, and Rance NE (2012). Role of kisspeptin/neurokinin B/dynorphin (KNDy) neurons in cutaneous vasodilation and the estrogen modulation of body temperature. Proceedings of the National Academy of Science, 109:19846-19851.

Morrow PKH, Mattair DN, and Hortobagyi GN (2011). Hot Flashes: A review of pathophysiology and treatment modalities. The Oncologist, 16:16581664.

Nakamura K and Morrison SF (2010). A thermosensory pathway mediating heat-defense responses. PNAS, 107:8848-8853.

Navarro VM (2013). Interactions between Kisspeptins and Neurokinin b. Advances in Experimental Medicine and Biology, 784:325-347.

Oakley AE, Steiner RA, Chavkin C, Clifton DK, Ferrara LK, and Reed SD (2015). [Kappa] agonists as a novel therapy for menopausal hot flashes. Menopause, Abstract May 18, 2015.

Rometo AM and Rance NE (2008). Changes in prodynorphin gene expression and neuronal morphology in the hypothalamus of postmenopausal women. Journal of Neuroendocrinology, 20:1376-1381.

Skorupskaite K, George JT, and Anderson RA (2014). The Kisspeptin-GnRH pathway in human reproductive health and disease. Human Reproduction Update, 4:485-500.

Uenoyama Y, Tsukamura H, and Maeda K (2014). KNDy neuron as a gatekeeper of puberty onset. The Journal of Obstetrics and Gynaecology Research, 40:1518-1526.

IS SOY A REMEDY FOR HOT FLASHES?

ConsumerLab.com 7/12/2011. Product Review; Menopause supplements (soy and Red Clover isoflavones, Black Cohosh) and progesterone creams.

Huang Y, Cao S, Nagamani M, Anderson KE, grady JJ, and Lu LJW (2005). Decreased circulating levels of tumor necrosis factor-a in postmenopausal women during consumption of soy-containing isoflavones. Journal of Clinical Endocrinology and Metabolism, 90 (7):3956-3962.

Jou HJ, Wu SC, Chang FW, Ling PY, Chu KS, and Wu WH (2008). Effect of intestinal production of equol on menopausal symptoms in women treated with soy isoflavones. International Journal of Gynaecology and Obstetrics, 102(1): 44-49.

Mense SM, Hei TK, Ganju RK, and Bhat HK (2008). Phytoestrogens and breast cancer prevention: Possible mechanisms of action. Environmental Health Perspectives, 116:426-433.

NAAMS (2011) Isoflavones Report/The role of soy isoflavones in menopausal health: Report of the North American Menopause Society/Wulf H. UTian Translational Science Symposium in Chicago IL. Menopause, 18:732-753.

OBESITY AND CARDIOVASCULAR RISK

IS ALL BODY FAT THE SAME?

Bird PJ (2006). Why does fat deposit on the hips and thighs of women and around the stomachs of men? Scientific American, May 15.

Hamdy O, Porramatikul S, and Al-Ozairi E (2006). Metabolic Obesity: the paradox between visceral and subcutaneous fat. Current Diabetes Reviews, 2:2-7.

Lovejoy JC, Champagne CM, de Jonge L, Xie H, and Smith SR (2008). Increased visceral fat and decreased energy expenditure during the menopausal transition. International Journal of Obesity, 32:949-958.

Matthews KA, Crawford SL, Chae CU, Everson-Rose SA, Sowers MF, Sternfeld B, and Sutton-Tyrrell K (2009). Are changes in cardiovascular disease risk factors in midlife women due to chronological aging or to the menopausal transition? Journal of the American College of Cardiology, 54:2366-2373.

Stolk RP, Meijer R, Mali W PTM, Grobbee DE, and van der Graaf Y (2003). Ultrasound measurements of intraabdominal fat estimate the metabolic syndrome better than do measurements of waist circumference. American Journal of Clinical Nutrition, 77:857-860.

Vasilescu M, Calota F, Balseanu TA, Cosma G, and Gragomir M (2011). Ultrasonographic measurement of intraabdominal adiposity, a simple method for screening and monitoring the metabolic Syndrome. World Academy of Science, Engineering and Technology, 59:790-794.

Zhu L, Yang Y, Xu P, Zou F, Yan X, Liao L, Xu J, O'Malley BW, and Xu Y (2013). Steroid Receptor Coactivator-1 mediates estrogenic actions to prevent body weight gain in female mice. Endocrinology, 154:150-154.

WHAT HAS ESTROGEN GOT TO DO WITH BELLY FAT?

Bird PJ (2006). Why does fat deposit on the hips and thighs of women and around the stomachs of men? Scientific American, May 15.

Di Carlo C, Tommaselli GA, Sammartino A, Bifulco G, Nasti A, and Nappi C (2004). Serum leptin levels and body composition in postmenopausal women: Effects of hormone therapy. Menopause, 11:466-473.

Hamdy O, Porramatikul S, and Al-Ozairi E (2006). Metabolic Obesity: The paradox between visceral and subcutaneous fat. Current Diabetes Reviews, 2:1-7.

Kohrt WM (2009). Exercise, weight gain and menopause. Medscape multispecialty, June 29, 2009.

Lobo RA (2008). Metabolic syndrome after menopause and the role of hormones. Maturitas, 60:10-18.

Lovejoy JC, Champagne CM, deJonge L, Xie H, and Smith SR (2008). Increased visceral fat and decreased energy expenditure during the menopausal transition. International Journal of Obesity, 32:949-958.

Salpeter SR, Walsh JM, Ormiston TM, Greyber E, Buckley NS, and Salpeter EE (2006). Meta-analysis: Effect of hormone-replacement therapy on components of the metabolic syndrome in postmenopausal women. Diabetes, Obesity, and Metabolism, 8:538-554.

Stolk RP, Meijer R, Mali WPTM, Grobbee DE, and van der Graaf Y (2003). Ultrasound measurements of intraabdominal fat estimate the metabolic syndrome better than do measurements of waist circumference. American Journal of Clinical Nutrition, 77:857-860.

Vasilescu M, Calota F, Balseanu TA, Cosma G, and Dragomir M (2011). Ultrasonographic measurement of intraabdominal adiposity: A simple method for screening and monitoring the metabolic syndrome. World Academy of Science, Engineering and Technology, 59:790-794.

Zhu L, Yang Y, Xu P, Xu P, Zou F, Yan X, Liao L, Xu J, O'Malley BW, and Xu Y (2013). Steroid Receptor Coactivator-1 mediates estrogenic actions to prevent body weight gain in female mice. Endocrinology, 154:150-158.

METABOLIC SYNDROME AND THE ROLE OF ESTROGEN

Belfiore A and Malaquarnera R (2011). Insulin Receptor and cancer. Endocrine-Related Cancer, 18:R125-R147.

Beilby J (2004). Definition of metabolic syndrome: Report of the national heart, lung, and blood institute/American Heart Association conference on scientific issues related to definition. Circulation, 109: 433-438.

Bird PJ (2006). Why does fat deposit on the hips and thighs of women and around the stomachs of men? Scientific American, May 15.

Di Carlo C, Tommaselli GA, Sammartino A, Bifulco G, Nasti A, and Nappi C (2004). Serum leptin levels and body composition in postmenopausal women: Effects of hormone therapy. Menopause, 11:466-473.

Hamdy O, Porramatikul S, and Al-Ozairi E (2006). Metabolic Obesity: The paradox between visceral and subcutaneous fat. Current Diabetes Reviews, 2:1-7.

Hilf R (1981). The actions of insulin as a hormonal factor in breast Cancer. Banbury Report, 8:317-337.

Hudis CA andGianni L (2011). Triple-negative breast cancer: An unmet medical need. The Oncologist, 16:1-11.

Kohrt WM (2009). Exercise, weight gain and menopause. Medscape Multispecialty, June 29, 2009.

Lobo RA (2008). Metabolic syndrome after menopause and the role of hormones. Maturitas, 60:10-18.

Lovejoy JC, Champagne CM, de Jonge L, Xie H, and Smith SR (2008). Increased visceral fat and decreased energy expenditure during the menopausal transition. International Journal of Obesity, 32:949-958.

Pollak MN (2007). Insulin, insulin like growth factor, insulin resistance and neoplasm. American Journal of Clinical Nutrition, 86:820s-822s.

Salpeter SR, Walsh JM, Ormiston TM, Greyber E, Buckley NS, and Salpeter EE (2006). Meta-analysis: Effect of hormone-replacement therapy on components of the metabolic syndrome in postmenopausal women. Diabetes Obesity Metabolism, 8:538-554.

Stachowiak G. Pertynski T, and Pertynska-Mapczewska M (2015). Metabolic Disorders in menopause. Przegląd Menopauzalny, 14:59-64.

Suba Z (2014). Triple negative breast cancer risk is defined by the defect in estrogen signaling: Prevention and therapeutic implications. Onco Targets and Therapy, 7:147-167.

MATTERS OF THE HEART

Chae CU and Derby CA (2011). The menopausal transition and cardiovascular risk. Obstetrics and Gynecology Clinics of North America, 38:477-488.

Dubey RK, Imthurn B, Barton M, and Jackson EK (2005). Vascular consequences of menopause and hormone therapy: Importance of timing of treatment and type of estrogen. Cardiovascular Research, 66:295-306.

Ferreri NR (2007). Estrogen-TNF interactions and vascular inflammation. American Journal of Physiology. Heart and Circulatory Physiology, 292:H2566-H2569.

Koenig W (2001). Inflammation and coronary heart disease: An overview. Cardiology in Review, 9:31-35.

Lobo RA (2008). Metabolic syndrome after menopause and the role of hormones. Maturitas, 60:10-18.

Manson JE, Hsia J, Johnson KC, Rossouw JE, Asaf AR, Lasser NL, Trevisan M, Black HR, Heckbert SR, Detrano R, Strickland OL, Wong ND, Crouse JR, Stein E, and Cushman M (2003). Estrogen plus progestin and the risk of coronary heart disease. New England Journal of Medicine, 349:523-534.

Matthews KA, Crawford SL, Chae CU, Everson-Rose SA, Sowers MF, Sternfeld B, and Sutton-Tyrrell K (2009). Are changes in cardiovascular disease due to chronological aging or to the menopausal transition? Journal of the American College of Cardiology, 54:2366-2373.

Pfeilschifter J, Koditz R, Pfoho M, and Schatz H (2002). Changes in proinflammatory cytokine activity after menopause. Endocrine Reviews, 23:90-119.

Rajsheker S, Manka D, Blomkains AL, Chatterjee TK, Stoll LL, and Weintraub NL (2010). Crosstalk between perivascular adipose tissue and blood vessels. Current Opinion in Pharmacology, 10:191-196.

Ridker PM, Hennekens CH, Buring JE, and Rifai N (2000). C-reactive protein and other markers of inflammation in the prediction of cardiovascular disease in women. New England Journal Medicine, 342:836-843.

Straub RH (2007). The complex role of estrogens in inflammation. <u>Endocrine Reviews</u>, 28:521-574.

Takao T, Kumagai C, Hisakawa N, Matsumoto R, and Hashimoto K (2005). Effect of 17B-estradiol on tumor necrosis factor-alpha-induced cytotoxicity in the human peripheral T lymphocytes. <u>Journal of Endocrinology</u>, 184:191197.

MENOPAUSE, METABOLISM, AND VISCERAL FAT ACCUMULATION

Batra A and Siegmund B (2012). The role of visceral fat. <u>Digestive Diseases</u>, 30:70-74.

Frayn KN (2000). Visceral fat and insulin-resistance-causative or correlative? <u>British Journal of Nutrition</u>, 83:s71-77.

Nielsen S, Guo Z, Johnson CM, Hensrud DD, and Jensen MD (2004). Splanchnic lipolysis in human obesity. <u>Journal of Clinical Investigation</u>, 113:1582-1588.

Kredel LI and Siegmund B (2014). Adipose-tissue and intestinal inflammation-visceral obesity and creeping fat. <u>Frontiers of Immunology</u>, 5:462-473.

Chistiakov DA, Bobryshev YV, Kozarov E, Sobenin IA, and Orekhov AN (2015). Role of gut microbiota in the modulation of atherosclerosisassociated immune response. <u>Frontiers in Microbiology</u>, 6:1-7.

Shuster A, Patlas M, Pinthus JH, and Mourtzakis M (2012). The clinical importance of visceral adiposity: A critical review of methods for visceral adipose tissue analysis. <u>British Journal of Radiology</u>, 85:1-10.

Yki-Jarvinen H (2010). Liver fat in the pathogenesis of insulin resistance and type 2 diabetes. <u>Digestive Diseases</u>, 28(1):203-209.

Klein S (2004). The case of visceral fat: Argument for the defense. <u>Journal of Clinical Investigation</u>, 11:1530-1532.

Lobo RA (2008). Metabolic syndrome after menopause and the role of hormones. <u>Maturitas</u>, 60:10-18.

Hanauer S (2005). Obesity and visceral fat: A growing inflammatory disease. <u>Nature Clinical Practice</u>. <u>Gastroenterology and Hepatology</u>. 2:245.

Kabir M, Catalano KJ, Ananthnarayan S, Kim SP, Van Citters GW, Dea MK, and Bergman RN (2005). Molecular evidence supporting the portal theory: A causative link between visceral adiposity and hepatic insulin resistance. <u>American Journal of Physiology</u>. <u>Endocrinology and Metabolism</u>, 288:E454E461.

Navarro VM and Kaiser UB (2013). Metabolic influences on neuroendocrine regulation of reproduction. Current Opinion in Endocrinology, Diabetes, and Obesity, 20:335-341.

Di Carlo C, Tommaselli GA, Sammartino A, Bifulco G, Nasti A, and Nappi C (2004). Serum leptin levels and body composition in postmenopausal women: effects of hormone therapy. Menopause, 11:466-473.

Hamdy O, Porramatikul S, and Al-Ozairi E (2006). Metabolic Obesity: The paradox between visceral and subcutaneous fat. Current Diabetes Reviews, 2:1-7.

Lovejoy JC, Champagne CM, deJonge L, Xie H, and Smith SR (2008). Increased visceral fat and decreased energy expenditure during the menopausal transition. International Journal of Obesity, 32:949-958.

Janssen I, Powell LH, Kazlauskaite R, and Dugan SA (2010). Testosterone and visceral fat in midlife women: the Study of Women's Health Across the Nation (SWAN) Fat Patterning Study. Obesity, 18:604-610.

Guthrie JR, Dennerstein L, Taffe JR, Ebeling PR, Randolph JF, Burger HG, and Wark JD (2003). Central abdominal fat and endogenous hormones during the menopausal transition. Fertility and Sterility, 79:1335-1340.

IMPACT OF VARIOUS BARIATRIC PROCEDURES IN TREATING DIABETES IN MENOPAUSE

Cummings DE, Overduin J, Foster-Schubert KE, and Carlson MJ (2007). Role of the bypassed proximal intestine in the anti-diabetic effects of bariatric surgery. Surgery for Obesity and Related Diseases, 3:109-115.

Rubino F (2008). Is type 2 diabetes an operable intestinal disease? A provocative yet reasonable hypothesis. Diabetes Care. 31:Suppl 2S290-296.

Vetter ML, Cardillo S, Rickels MR, and Izbal N (2009). Narrative review: Effect of Bariatric Surgery on type 2 diabetes mellitus. Annals of Internal Medicine, 150:94-103.

BONE HEALTH: WHAT'S MENOPAUSE GOT TO DO WITH IT?

Belson DT and Cummings SR (2005). Aromatose Inhibitors and the syndrome of arthralgias with estrogen deprivation. Arthritis and Rheumatism, 52:2594-2598.

Cenci S, Toraldo G, Neale Weitzmann M, Roggia C, Gao Y, Qian WP, Sierra O, and Pacifici R (2003). Estrogen deficiency induces bone loss by increasing T cell proliferation and lifespan through IFN-alpha induced class II transactivator. Proceedings of the National Academies of Sciences of the United States of America, 100:10405-10410.

Kennel KA and Drake MT (2009). Adverse effects of bisphosphonates: Implications for osteoporosis management. Mayo Clinic Proceedings, 84:632-638.

Murray RK and Gross PL (2012). Biochemical case histories: Osteoporosis (Chapter 57). In: M Weitz and B Kearns, (Eds.). Harper's Illustrated Biochemistry, (Ed. 29). New York: McGraw Hill.

Siefert-Klauss V and Prior JC (2010). Progesterone and bone: Actions promoting bone health in women. Journal of Osteoporosis, ID 845180.

Vam Beel E. Lowik C, Van Der Pluijm G, and Papapoulos S (1999). The role of geranylgeranylation in bone resorption and its suppression by bisphosphonates in fetal bone explants in vitro: a clue to the mechanism of action of nitrogen-containing bisphosphonates. Journal of Bone and Mineral Research, 14:722-729.

Yasuda H, Shima N, Nakagawa N, Mochizuki S-I, Yano K, Fujise N, Sato Y, Goto M, Yamaguchi K, Kuriyama M, Kanno T, Murakami A, Tsuda E, Morinaga T, and Higashio K (1998). Identify of osteoclastogenesis inhibitory factor (OCIF) and osteoprotegerin (OPG): A mechanism by which OPG/OCIF inhibits osteoclastogenesis in vitro. Endocrinology, 139:13291337.

THE VALUE OF MONITORING BONE HEALTH WITH AGING

Blake GM, Fogelman I. The role of DXA bone density scans in the diagnosis and treatment of osteoporosis. Postgrad Med J (2007) 83; 509-517.

Clarke b. Normal bone anatomy and physiology. Cl J Am Soc Neurol (2008) 3; S131-139.

Garnero P, Sornay-Rendu E, Claustrat B, Delmas PD. Biochemical markers of bone turnover, endogenous hormones and the risk of fractures in postmenopausal women: the OFELY study. J of bone and Mineral Research (2000) 15; 1526-1536.

Marini F, Cianferotti L, Brandi ML. Epigenetic mechanisms in bone biology and osteoporosis; can they drive therapeutic choices. International J Mol Sciences (2016) 17; 1329-1338.

Metcalfe D. The pathophysiology of osteoporotic hip fracture. MJM (2008) 11;51-57.

Kanis JA, McCloskey EV, Johansson H, Oden A, Melton LJ 111, Khaltaev N. A reference standard for the description of osteoporosis. Bone (2008) 42; 467-475.

Management of osteoporosis in postmenopausal women: 2010 position statement of the North American Menopause Society. Menopause (2010) 17; 25-54.

Panula J, Pihlajamaki H, Mattila VM, Jaatinen P, Vahlberg T, Aarnio P, Kivela S-L. Mortality and cause of death in hip fracture patients aged 65 or older- a population-based study. Musculoskeletal disorders (2011) 12; 105-111.

Schnell S, Friedman SM, Mendelson DA, Bingham KW, Kates SL. The 1-year mortality of patients treated in a hip fracture program for elders. Geriatric Orthopaedic Surgery and Rehab (2010) 1; 6-14.

Schuit SC, van der Klift M, Weel AE, de Laet CE, Burger H, Seeman E, Hofman A, Uitterlinden AG, van leeuwen JP, Pols HA. Fracture incidence and association with bone mineral density in elderly men and women: the Rotterdam Study. Bone (2004) 34; 195-202.

Watts NB, The fracture risk assessment tool (FRAX) : applications in clinical practice. J Womens Health (Larchmt) (2011) 4; 525-31.

Wheater G, Elshahaly M, Tuck SP, Datta HK, van Laar J. The clinical utility of bone marker measurements in osteoporosis. J of Translational Medicine (2013) 11; 201 – 215.

Wu T. Hologic bone densitometry and the evolution of DXA. Hologic Asia Pacific Hologic, Inc. (2012) Bedford, Mass.

DOCTOR, WHY DOES IT HURT DOWN THERE?

Baumgart J, Nilsson K, Evers AS, Kallak, TK, and Poromaa IS (2013). Sexual dysfunction in women on adjuvant endocrine therapy after breast cancer. Menopause, 20:162-168.

Boskey ER, Cone RA, Whaley KJ, and Moench TR (2001). Origins of vaginal acidity: High D/L lactate ratio is consistent with bacteria being the primary source. Human Reproduction, 16:1809-1813.

Editorial Vaginal Dialogues (2014). Menopause, 21:437.

Kendall A, Dowsett M, FolkerdE, and Smith I (2006). Caution: Vaginal estradiol appears to be contraindicated in postmenopausal women on adjuvant aromatase inhibitors. Annals of Oncology, 17:584-587.

Pfeiler G, Glatz C, Königsberg R, Geisendorfer T, Fink-Retter A, Kubista E, Singer CF, and Seifert M (2011). Vaginal estriol to overcome side-effects of aromatase inhibitors in breast cancer patients. Climacteric, 14:339-344.

MENOPAUSAL INTIMACY: WHAT'S SEX GOT TO DO WITH IT?

Basson R (2010). Testosterone therapy for reduced libido in women. Therapeutic Advances in Endocrinology and Metabolism, 1:155-164.

Boskey ER, Cone RA, Whaley KJ, and Moench TR (2001). Origin of vaginal acidity: High D/L lactate ration is consistent with bacteria being the primary source. Human Reproduction, 16:1809-1813.

Carley ME, Rickard DJ, Gebhart JB, Webb MJ, Podratz KC, and Spelsberg TC (2003). Distribution of estrogen receptors alpha and beta mRNA I mouse urogenital tissues and their expression after oophorectomy and estrogen replacement. International Urogynecology Journal and Pelvic Floor Dysfunction, 14:141-145.

Goldey KL and vanAnders SM (2011). Sexy thoughts: Effects of sexual cognitions on testosterone, cortisol, and arousal in women. Hormones and Behavior, 59:754-764.

Greenwel P, Tanaka S, Penkov D, Zhang W, Olive M, Moll J, Vinson C, Di Liberto M, and Ramirez F (2000). Tumor necrosis factor alpha inhibits type 1 collagen synthesis through repressive CCAAT/enhancer-binding proteins. Molecular and Cellular Biology, 20:912-918.

Shifren JL (2015). Testosterone for midwife women: The hormone of desire? NAMS Practice Pearl, 1-5.

Simunic V, Banovic I, Ciglar S, Jeren L, Pavicic Baldani D, and Sprem M (2003). Local estrogen treatment in patients with urogenital symptoms. International Journal of Gynecology and Obstretics, 82:187-197.

Stevenson S and Thronton J (2007). Effect of estrogens on skin aging and the potential role of SERMS. Clinical Interventions in Aging, 2:283-297.

Tan O, Bradshaw K, and Carr B (2012). Management of vulvovaginal atrophy-related sexual dysfunction in postmenopausal women. Menopause, 19:109-117.

LET'S TALK ABOUT TESTOSTERONE

Basson R. Testosterone therapy for reduced libido in women. Endocrinology and Metabolism (2010) 1; 155-164.

Basson R. Rees P, R Wang, Montegto AL, Incrocci L. Sexual function in chronic illness. J Sex Med (2010) 7;374-88.

Bennett NC, Garcliner RA, Hoper JD, Johnson DW, Gobe GC, Internal J of Biochem and Cell Biology (2010) 42; 813-827.

Burger HG, Dudley EC, Cui J, Dennerstein L, Hopper JL. A prospective longitudinal study of serum testosterone, dehydroepiandrosterone sulfate and sex-binding globulin levels through the menopause transition. J Cl Endocrin Metab (2000) 85;2832-8.

Davis SA, Davison SL. Current perspectives on testosterone therapy for women. Menopause Medium (2012) 20;51-54.

Channer KS, Jones TH. Cardiovascular effects of testosterone: implications of the "male menopause." October 20, 2015 HTTP://heart.BMJ.com.

Gao W, Bohl CE, Dalton JT. Chemistry and structural biology of androgen receptors. Chem Rev (2005) 105; 3352-3370.

Glaser R, Dimitrakakis C. Testosterone therapy in women; myths and misconceptions. Maturitas (2013) 74;230-39.

George AJ. The actions and side effects of anabolic steroids in sport and social abuse. Andrologie (2003) 13; 354-366.

Goldey KL, Van Anders SM. Sexy thoughts; effects of sexual cognition on testosterone, cortisol and arousal in women. Hormones and Behavior (2011) 50;754-764.

Griggs RC, Kingston W, Jozefowicz RF, Herr BE, Forbes G, Halliday D. Effect of testosterone on muscle mass and muscle protein synthesis. J Appl. Physiol (1989) 66;498-503.

Lamb DR. Anabolic steroids in athletics: how well do they work and how dangerous are they? Am J. Sports Med (1984) 12;31-38.

Morley MD, Perry HM. Androgens and women at the menopause and beyond. J Gerontology (2003) 58A; 409-416.

Rohr UD. The impact of testosterone imbalance on depression and women's health. Maturitas (2002) 15; 525-46.

Shifren JL. NAMS Practice Pearl. June 24, 2015.

Shufelt CL, Braunstein GD. Safety of testosterone use in women. Maturitas (2009) 63; 63-66.

DO WOMEN NEED THEIR OWN "VIAGRA"?

Basson R (2010). Testosterone therapy for reduced libido in women. Therapeutic Advances in Endocrinology and Metabolism, 1(4):155-164.

Borsini F, Evans K, Jason K, Rohde F, Alexander B, and Pollentier S (2002). Pharmacology of flibanserin. CNS Drug Reviews, 8(2):117-142.

Burger HG, Dudley EC, Cui J, Dennerstein L, and Hopper JL (2000). A prospective longitudinal study of serum testosterone, dehydroepiandrosterone sulfate, and sex hormone-binding globulin levels through the menopause transition. Journal of Clinical Endocrinology and Metabolism, 85(8):2832-2839.

Davis SR and Davison SL (2012). Current perspectives on testosterone therapy for women. Menopause Medicine, 20:S1-S4.

Drug Safety and Risk Management Advisory Commmittee (2015). Flibanserin for the Treatment of Hypoactive Sexual Desire Disorder in Premenopausal Women NDA 022526 Advisory Committee Briefing Document 4 June 2015, i-v.

Glaser R and Dimitrakakis C (2013). Testosterone therapy in women: Myths and misconceptions. Maturitas, 74:230-234.

Morley JE and Perry HM (2003). Androgens and women at the menopause and beyond. Journal of Gerontology, 58:409-416.

Nappi RI, Martini E, Terreno E, Albani F, Santamaria V, Tonani S, Chiovato L, and Polatti F (2010). Management of hypoactive sexual desire disorder in women: Current and emerging therapies. International Journal of Women's Health, 2:167-175.

Nurnberg HG, Hensley PL, Heiman JR, Croft HA, Debattista C, and Paine S (2008). Sildenafil treatment of women with antidepressant-associated sexual dysfunction. Journal of the American Medical Association, 300:395404.

Pfaus JG (1999). Neurobiology of sexual behavior. Current Opinion in Neurobiology, 9:751-758.

Schwenkhagen A and Studd J (2009). Role of Testosterone in the treatment of hypoactive sexual desire disorder. Maturitas, 63:152-159.

Sobecki JN, Curlin FA, Rasinski KA, and Lindau ST (2012). What we don't talk about when we don't talk about sex: Results of a national survey of U.S. obstetrician/gynecologists. Journal of Sexual Medicine, 9:1285-1294.

A BRIEF HISTORY OF NONSURGICAL TREATMENTS OF STRESS URINARY INCONTINENCE

Bo K, Talseth T, and Holme I (1999). Single blind, randomized controlled trial of pelvic floor exercises, electrical stimulation, vaginal cones, and no treatment in management of genuine stress incontinence in women. BMJ, 318:487-493.

Chancellor MB (2001). First-line therapy for stress incontinence. Reviews in Urology, 2:229-230.

Bordman R (2007). Pessary insertion. Canadian Family Physician, 53:424425.

Cody JD, Richardson K, Moehrer B, Hextall A, and Glazener CM (2009). Oestrogen therapy for urinary incontinence in post-menopausal women. Cochrane Database of Systematic Reviews, (4):CD001405.

Daneshgari F and Moore C (2006). Advancing the understanding of pathophysiological rationale for the treatment of stress urinary incontinence in women: the "trampoline theory." BJU International, 98:814.

DuBeau CE (2005). Estrogen treatment for urinary incontinence: Never, now, or in the future? Journal of the American Medical Association, 293:998-1001.

Fantl JA, Bump RC, Robinson D, McClish DK, and Wyman JF (1996). Efficacy of estrogen supplementation in the treatment of urinary incontinence. Obstetrics and Gynecology, 88:745-749.

Kegel, AH (1948). The nonsurgical treatment of genital relaxation. Annals of Western Medicine and Surgery, 31:213-216.

Kegel AH (1948). Progressive resistance exercise to the functional restoration of the perineal muscles. <u>American Journal of Obstetrics and</u> and Gynecology, 56:238-248.

Jones KA and Harmanli O (2010). Pessary use in pelvic organ prolapse and urinary incontinence. <u>Reviews in Obstetrics and Gynecology</u>, 3:3-9.

Weber MA, Kleijn MH, Langendam M, Limpens J, Heineman MJ, and Roovers JP (2015). Local oestogen for pelvic floor disorders: A systematic review. <u>PLOS ONE</u>, 10; e0136265.

DOES ESTROGEN HELP SKIN AGE BETTER?

Creidi P and Faivre B (1994). Effect of a conjugated oestrogen (Premarin) cream on aging facial skin. A comparative study with a placebo cream. <u>Maturitas</u>, 19; 211-223.

Fuchs KO, Solis O, Tapawan R, and Paranjpe J (2003). The effects of an estrogen and glycolic acid cream on the facial skin of postmenopausal women. <u>Cutis</u>, 71:481-488.

Greenwel P, Shizuko T, Penkov D, Zhang W, Olive M, Moll J, Vinson C, Diliberto M, and Ramirez F (2000). Tumor Necrosis Factor Alpha Inhibits Type 1 collagen synthesis through repressive CCAAT/Enhancer-Binding Proteins. <u>Molecular and Cellular Biology</u>, 20:912-918.

Hess H (2008). <u>The perfect Menopause: Seven steps to the best time of your life</u>. Rochester: Westfall Park Publishing Group.

Kainz C, Gitsch G, Stani J, Breitenecker G, Binder M, and Schmidt JB (1993). When applied to facial skin, does estrogen ointment have systemic effects? <u>Archives of Gynecology and Obstetrics</u>, 253:71-74.

Schmidt JB, Binder M, Demschik G, Bieglmayer C, and Reiner A (1996). Treatment of skin aging with topical estrogens. <u>International Journal of Dermatology</u>, 35:669-674.

Stevenson S and Thornton J (2007). Effect of estrogens on skin aging and the potential role of SERMS. <u>Clinical Interventions in Aging</u>, 2:283-297.

Thornton MJ (2013). Estrogen and aging skin. <u>Dermato-Endocrinology</u>, 5:264-270.

HAIR TODAY: GONE TOMORROW.
WHAT'S TESTOSTERONE GOT TO DO WITH IT?

Glaser RL, Dimitrakakis C, and Messenger AG (2012). Improvement in scalp hair growth in androgen-deficient women treated with testosterone: A questionnaire study. The British Journal of Dermatology, 166:274-278.

Price VH (2003). Androgenetic alopecia in women. Journal of Investigative Dermatology Symposium Proceedings, 8:24-27.

Worth T (2011). Hair loss health Center; Women and hair loss; possible causes. Retrieved May 24, 2016 from http://www.webmd.com/skinproblems-and-treatments/hair-loss/features/women-hair-loss-causes

MOODS AND MEMORY

MOODS AND MENOPAUSE

Craig MC, Maki PM, and Murphy DG (2005). The Women's Health Initiative Memory Study: Findings and implications for treatment. The Lancet. Neurology, 4:190-194.

Douma SL, Husband C, O'Donnell ME, Barwin BN, and Woodend AK (2005). Estrogen-related mood disorders: Reproductive life cycle factors. 28:364375.

Douma SL, Husband C, O'Donnell ME, Barwin BN, and Woodend AK (2005). Estrogen-related mood disorders. Advances in Nursing Science, 28:364375.

Holschneider DP, Kumazawa T, Hen K, and Shih JC (1998). Tissue-Specific effects of estrogen on monoamine oxidase A and B in the rat. Life Sciences, 63:155-160.

LeBlanc ES, Janowsky J, Chan BK, and Nelson HD (2001). Hormone replacement therapy and cognition: Systematic review and meta-analysis. Journal of the American Medical Association, 285:1489-1499.

Lokuge S, Frey BN, Foster JA, Soares CN, and Steiner M (2011). Depression in women: Windows of vulnerability and new insights into the link between estrogen and serotonin. Journal of Clinical Psychiatry, 72: e1563e1569.

Morrison JH, Brinton RD, Schmidt PJ, and Gore AC (2006). Estrogen, menopause, and the aging brain: How basic neuroscience can inform hormone therapy in women. Journal of Neuroscience, 26:10332-10348.

Morrison JH (2008). Unraveling the estrogen paradox: When is estrogen good for the brain? Advances in Brain Research, 1-3.

Murphy DD, Cole NB, Greenberger V, and Segal M (1998). Estradiol increases dendritic spine density by reducing GABA neurotransmission in hippocampal neurons. Journal of Neuroscience, 18:2550-2559.

Shepherd JE (2001). Effects of estrogen on cognition, mood, and degenerative brain diseases. Journal of the American Pharmaceutical Association, 41:2-16.

Shumaker Sa, Reboussin BA, Espeland MA, Rapp SR, McBee WL, Dailey M, Bowen D, Terrell T, and Jones BN (1998). The Women's Health Initiative Memory Study (WHIMS): A trial of the effect of estrogen therapy in preventing and slowing the progression of dementia. Controlled Clinical Trials, 19:604-621.

Woolley CS (2007). Acute effects of estrogen on neuronal physiology. 47:657-680.

PANIC ATTACK OR GENERALIZED ANXIETY DISORDER?

Bouton ME, MIneka S, and Barlow DH (2001). A modern learning theory perspective on the etiology of panic disorder. Psychological Review, 108:432.

Lacasse JR and Leo J (2005). Serotonin and depression: A disconnect between the advertisements and the scientific literature. PLOS Medicine, 2:E392-E398.

Leicht G, Mulert C, Eser D, Samann PG, Ertl M, Laenger A, Karch S, Pogarell O, Meindl T, Czisch M, and Rupprecht R (2013). Benzodiazepines counteract rostral anterior cingulated cortex activation induced by cholecystokinin-tetrapeptide in humans. Biological Psychiatry, 73:337-344.

Maddock R (2010). Panic Attacks as a problem of pH. Scientific American, May 18.

Martinez JM and Marangell LB (2006). Psychiatric Disorders (Chapter 23). In: MC Gurtis, S Overhold, and MP Hopkins, (Eds.). Glass' Office Gynecology (Ed. 6). Philadelphia: Lippincott Williams & Wilkins, 578-600.

Moret C and Briley M (2011). The importance of norepinephrine in depression. Neuropsychiatric Disease and Treatment, 7:9-13.

Wemmie JA, Taugher RJ, and Kreple CJ (2013). Acid-sensing ion channels in pain and disease. Nature Reviews/Neuroscience, 14:461-471.

IS THERE A WINDOW FOR MENOPAUSAL HORMONE REPLACEMENT THERAPY TO HELP REDUCE THE RISK OF DEMENTIA?

Birge SJ. Alzheimer's disease research: possible causes, potential treatment. Poster Book (1996) American Academy of Family Physicians, New Orleans.

Cummings JL, Benson DF, Hill MA. Aphasia in dementia of Alzheimer's type. Neurology (1985) 35;394-397.

Coker LH, Espeland MA, Rapp SR, Legault C, Resnick SM, Hogan P, Gaussoin S, Dailey M, Shumaker SA. Postmenopausal hormone therapy and cognitive outcomes: the Women's Health Initiative Memory Study (WHIMS). Journal of Steroid biochemistry and Molecular Biology (2010) 118; 304-310.

Craig MC, Murphy DG. The Women's Health Initiative Memory Study: findings and implications for treatment. Lancet//Neurology (2005) 4; 190-194 .

Henderson VW. Cognitive changes after menopause: influence of estrogen. Cl ObGyn (2008) 51;618-26.

Jacobs E, D'Esposito M. Estrogen shapes dopamine-dependent cognitive processes: implications for women's health. The Journal of Neuroscience (2011) 31; 5286-5293.

LeBlanc ES, Janowsky J, Nelson HD. Hormone replacement and cognition. systematic review and meta analysis. JAMA (2001) 21; 285; 1489-99.

Lokuge S, Grey BN, Foster JA, Soares CN, Steiner M. Depression in women: window of vulnerability and new insights into the link between estrogen and serotonin. J Cl Psych. (2011) 72;e1563-e1569.

Shepherd JE. Effects of Estrogen on cognition, mood, and degenerative brain diseases. J Am Pharm Assoc (2001) 41: (2) 1-12.

Shumaker SA, Reboussin BA, Espeland MA, Rapp SR, McBee WL, Dailey M, Bowen D, Terrell T, Jones BN. The Women's Health Initiative Memory Study (WHIMS): a trial of the effect of estrogen therapy in preventing and slowing the progression of dementia. Controlled Clinical Trials (1998) 19; 604-621 Pub Elsevier Science Inc, NY, NY.

Simpkins JW, Perez E, Wang X, Yang S, Wen Y, Singh M. The potential for estrogens in preventing Alzheimer's disease and vascular dementia. Ther Adv Neurol Disord (2009) 2; 31-49.

Singh M, Meyer EM, Millard WJ, Simpkins JW. Ovarian steroid deprivation results in a reversible learning impairment and compromised cholinergic function in female Sprague-Dawley rats. Brain Research (1994) 644;305-312.

Toran-Allerand CD, Miranda RC, Benthaam WDL, Sohrabji F, Trown RTJ, Hochberg RB, MacLusky NJ. Estrogen receptors co-localize with low-affinity nerve growth factor receptors in cholinergic neurons of the basal forebrain. Proc Natl Acad Sci (1992) 89;4668-4672.

BREAST CANCER

ESTROGEN AND BREAST CANCER: A LOVE-HATE RELATIONSHIP

Allen E and Diosy AE (1923). An ovarian hormone; preliminary report on its localization, ex traction and partial purification and action in test animals. Journal of the American Medical Association, 81:819-821.

Beatson GT (1896). On the treatment of inoperable causes of carcinoma of the mammary: Suggestions for a new method of treatment with illustrative cases. Lancet, 2:104.

Dawood S and Cristofanilli M (2007). Endocrine resistance in breast cancer: What really matters? Annals of Oncology, 18:1289-1291.

Haddo WR, Wilkinson JM, Paterson E, and Koller PC (1944). Influence of synthetic estrogens upon advanced malignant disease. BMJ, 2:393.

Haldosen L-A, Zhao C, and Dahlman-Wright K (2013). Estrogen receptor beta in breast cancer. Molecular and Cellular Endocrinology, 382:665-672.

Jordan VC (2014). Another scientific strategy to prevent breast cancer in postmenopausal women by enhancing estrogen-induced apoptosis. Menopause, 10:1160-1164.

Jordan VC and Ford LG (2011). Paradoxical clinical effect of estrogen on breast cancer risk: A "new" biology of estrogen-induced apoptosis. Cancer Prevention Research, 4:633-637.

Labrie F, Luu-The V, Labrie C, Belanger A, Simard J, Lin S-X, and Pelletier G (2003). Endocrine and intracrine sources of androgens in women: Inhibition of breast cancer and other roles of androgens and their precursor dehydroepiandrosterone. Endocrine Reviews, 24:152-182.

Lathrop AEC and Loeb L (1916). Further investigations on the origin of tumors in mice. 111. On the part played by internal secretions in the spontaneous development of tumors. Journal of Can Research, 1-19.

Lees JC (1937). The inhibition of growth by 1.2:5.6 Dibenzanthracene and other agents. Quarterly Journal of Experimental Physiology, 27:161-170.

Love RR and Philips J (2002). Oophorectomy for breast cancer: History revisited. Journal of the National Cancer Institute, 94:1433-1434.

Melisko ME, Goldman M, and Rugo H (2010). Amelioration of sexual adverse effects in the early breast cancer patient. Journal of Cancer Survivorship, 4:247-255.

Mense SM, Remotti F, Bhan A, Singh B, El-Tamer M, Kei TK, and Bhat HR (2008). Estrogen-induced breast cancer: Alterations in breast morphology and oxidative stress as a function of estrogen exposure. Toxicology and Applied Pharmacology, 232:78-85.

Obiorah I and Jordan VC (2013). Scientific rationale for postmenopause delay in the use of conjugated equine estrogens among postmenopausal women that causes reduction in breast cancer incidence and mortality. Menopause, 20:372-382.

Osborne CK and Schiff R (2005). Estrogen-receptor biology: Continuing progress and therapeutic implications. Journal of Clinical Oncology, 23:1616-1622.

Writing Group for the Women's Health Initiative Investigators (2002). Risks and Benefits of estrogen plus progestin in healthy postmenopausal women. Journal of the American Medical Association, 288-321.

Yager JD and Davidson NE (2013). Estrogen carcinogenesis in breast cancer. New England Journal of Medicine, 354:270-282.

Yager JD (2000). Endogenous estrogens as carcinogens through metabolic activation. Journal of the National Cancer Institute Monographs, 27:67-73.

Zhang Q, Aft RL, and Gross ML (2008). Estrogen carcinogenesis: Specific identification of estrogen-modified nucleobase in breast tissue from women. Chemical Research in Toxicology, 21:1509-1513.

IS ALL BREAST CANCER THE SAME?

Allen E and Diosy AE (1923). An ovarian hormone: Preliminary report on its localization, ex traction and partial purification and action in test animals. Journal of the American Medical Association, 81:819.

Beatson GT (1896). On the treatment of inoperable causes of carcinoma of the mammary: Suggestions for a new method of treatment with illustrative cases. Lancet, 2:104.

Belfiore A (2011). Malaguarnera R+. Insulin receptor and cancer. <u>Endocrine-Related Cancer</u>, 18:R125-R147.

Dawood S and Cristofanilli M (2007). Endocrine resistance in breast cancer: What really matters. <u>Annals of Oncology</u>, 18:1289-1291.

Dunn BK, Agurs-Collins T, Browne D, Lubet R, and Johnson KA (2010). Health disparities in breast cancer: Biology meets socioeconomic status. <u>Breast Cancer Research and Treatment</u>, 121:281-292.

Haddo WR, Wilkinson JM, Paterson E, and Koller PC (1944). Influence of synthetic estrogens upon advanced malignant disease. <u>BMJ</u>, 2:393.

Hilf R, Livingston JN, and Crofton DH (1988). Effects of diabetes and sex steroid hormones on insulin receptor tyrosine kinase activity in R3230AC mammary adenocarcinomas. <u>Cancer Research</u>, 48:3742-3750.

Hilf R (1981). The actions of insulin as a hormonal factor in breast cancer. <u>Banbury Report 8 in Hormones and Breast Cancer</u>, Cold Spring Harbor Laboratory. 317-337.

Hudis CA and Gianni L (2011). Triple-negative breast cancer: An unmet medical need. <u>The Oncologist</u>, 16:1-11.

Jordan VC (2014). Another scientific strategy to prevent breast cancer in postmenopausal women by enhancing estrogen-induced apoptosis. <u>Menopause</u>, 10:1160-1164.

Jordan VC and Ford LG (2011). Paradoxical Clinical Effect of Estrogen on Breast Cancer Risk: A "new" biology of estrogen-induced apoptosis. <u>Cancer Prevention Research</u>, 4:633-637.

Lees JC (1937). The inhibition of growth by 1.2:5.6 Dibenzanthracene and other agents. <u>Quarterly Journal of Experimental Physiology</u>, 27:161-170.

Love RR and Philips J (2002). Oophorectomy for breast cancer: History revisited. <u>Journal of the National Cancer Institute</u>, 94:1433-1434.

Maiti B, Kundranda MN, Spiro TP, and Daw HA (2010). The association of metabolic syndrome with triple-negative breast cancer. <u>Breast Cancer Research and Treatment</u>, 121:479-483.

Obiorah I and Jordan VC (2013). Scientific rationale for postmenopause delay in the use of conjugated equine estrogens among postmenopausal women that causes reduction in breast cancer incidence and mortality. <u>Menopause</u>, 20:372-382.

Osborne CK and Schiff R (2005). Estrogen-receptor biology: Continuing progress and therapeutic implications. <u>Journal of Clinical Oncology</u>, 23:1616-1622.

Pollak MN (2007). Insulin, insulin-like growth factors, insulin resistance, and neoplasia. <u>American Journal of Clinical Nutrition</u>, 86:820S-822S.

Suba Z (2014). Triple negative breast cancer risk is defined by the defect in estrogen signaling: Prevention and therapeutic implications. <u>Onco Targets and Therapy</u>, 7:147-167.

Yager JD and Davidson NE (2006). Estrogen carcinogenesis in breast cancer. <u>New England Journal of Medicine</u>, 354:270-282.

Yager JD (2000). Endogenous estrogens as carcinogens through metabolic activation. <u>Journal of the National Cancer Institute. Monographs</u>. 27:67-73.

Zhang Z, Wang J, Tacha DE, Li P, Bremer RE, Chen H, Wei B, Xiao X, Da J, Skinner K, Hicks DG, Bu H. and Tang T (2014). Folate receptor alpha associated with triple-negative breast cancer and poor prognosis. <u>Archives of Pathology and Laboratory Medicine</u>, 138:890-895.

BRCA GENES: PROTECTOR FROM OR CAUSE OF BREAST CANCER?

Brandt-Rauf S, Raveis VH, Drummond NF, Conte JA, and Rothman SM (2006). Ashkenazi Jews and breast cancer: The consequences of linking ethnic identity to genetic disease. <u>American Journal of Public Health</u>, 96:1979-1988.

Deng C-X and Wang RH (2003). Roles of BRCA1 in DNA damage repair-a link between development and cancer. <u>Human Molecular Genetics</u>, 12:R1131123.

Murray RK, Granner DK, Mayes PA, and Rodwell VW (2000). DNA organization, replication, and repair (Chapter 38). In: <u>Harper's Illustrated Biochemistry, (Ed. 22)</u>. Stamford: Appleton and Lange, 412-434.

National Cancer Institute. BRCA1 and BRCA2: cancer risk and genetic testing. April 1, 2015.

Yoshida K and Miki Y (2004). Role of BRCA1 and BRCA2 as regulators of DNA repair, transcription, and cell cycle in response to DNA damage. <u>Cancer Science</u>. 95:866-871.

Wu J, Lu L-Y, and Yu X (2010). The role of BRCA1 in DNA damage response. <u>Protein Cell</u>, 1:117-123.

INTIMACY AND THE BREAST CANCER SURVIVOR

Course JF, LIndzey J, Grandien K, Gustafsson J-A, and Korach KS (1997). Tissue distribution and quantitative analysis of estrogen receptor-alpha (ER alpha) and estrogen receptor-beta (ER beta) messenger ribonucleic acid in the wild-type and ER alpha knockout mouse. Endocrinology, 138:46134621.

Dew JE, Wren BG, and Eden JA (2003). A cohort study of topical vaginal estrogen therapy in women previously treated for breast cancer. Climacteric, 6:45-52.

Kendall A. Dowsett M, Folkerd E, and Smith I (2006). Caution: Vaginal estradiol appears to be contraindicated in postmenopausal women on adjuvant aromatase inhibitors. Annals of Oncology, 17:584-587.

Labrie F, Archer D, Bouchard C, Fortier M, Cusan L, Gomez JL, Girard G, Baron M, Ayotte N, Moreau M, Dube R, Cote I, Labrie C, Lavoie L, Berger L,

Gilbert L, Martel C, and Balser J (2009). Intravaginal dehydroepiandrosterone (Prasterone), a physiological and highly efficient treatment of vaginal atrophy. Menopause, 16:907-922.

Melisko ME, Goldman M, and Rugo HS (2010). Amelioration of sexual adverse effects in the early breast cancer patient. Journal of Cancer Survivorship, 4:247-255.

Tan O, Bradshaw K, and Carr BR (2012). Management of vulvovaginal atrophy-related sexual dysfunction in postmenopausal women. Menopause, 19:109-117.

Witherby S, Johnson J, Demers L, Mount S, Littenberg B, Maclean CK, Wood M, and Muss H (2011). Topical Testosterone for breast cancer patients with vaginal atrophy related to aromatase inhibitors: A phase 1/11 study. The Oncologist, 16:424-431.